DYSLEXIA UNLOCKED

DYSLEXIA UNLOCKED

How to be successful in work and life

Natalie Brooks

GREEN TREE
LONDON · OXFORD · NEW YORK · NEW DELHI · SYDNEY

GREEN TREE
Bloomsbury Publishing Plc
50 Bedford Square, London, WC1B 3DP, UK
Bloomsbury Publishing Ireland Limited,
29 Earlsfort Terrace, Dublin 2, D02 AY28, Ireland

BLOOMSBURY, GREEN TREE and the Green Tree logo
are trademarks of Bloomsbury Publishing Plc

First published in Great Britain 2026

Copyright © Natalie Brooks, 2026

Natalie Brooks has asserted her right under the Copyright,
Designs and Patents Act, 1988, to be identified as Author of this work

For legal purposes the Acknowledgements on p. 264
constitute an extension of this copyright page

All rights reserved. No part of this publication may be: i) reproduced or transmitted in any form, electronic or mechanical, including photocopying, recording or by means of any information storage or retrieval system without prior permission in writing from the publishers; or ii) used or reproduced in any way for the training, development or operation of artificial intelligence (AI) technologies, including generative AI technologies. The rights holders expressly reserve this publication from the text and data mining exception as per Article 4(3) of the Digital Single Market Directive (EU) 2019/790

Bloomsbury Publishing Plc does not have any control over, or responsibility for, any third-party websites referred to or in this book. All internet addresses given in this book were correct at the time of going to press. The author and publisher regret any inconvenience caused if addresses have changed or sites have ceased to exist, but can accept no responsibility for any such changes

A catalogue record for this book is available from the British Library
Library of Congress Cataloguing-in-Publication data has been applied for

ISBN: TPB: 978-1-3994-2657-2; ePUB: 978-1-3994-2659-6; ePDF: 978-1-3994-2658-9

2 4 6 8 10 9 7 5 3 1

Typeset in Aestetico by Lumina Datamatics Ltd
Printed and bound in Great Britain by Clays Ltd, Elcograf S.p.A.

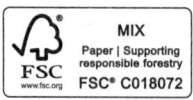

To find out more about our authors and books visit www.bloomsbury.com
and sign up for our newsletters

For product safety related questions contact productsafety@bloomsbury.com

Contents

Introduction	1
1. Understanding dyslexia	11
2. Dyslexic traits	19
Section One: Unlocking dyslexic confidence	**40**
3. Understanding why dyslexia impacts confidence	43
4. How to grow in confidence	59
5. Maintaining confidence in the long term	87
Section Two: Unlocking dyslexic strategies	**94**
6. How to get the most out of the strategies	97
7. How to talk about dyslexia with others	105
8. Tiredness	115
9. Working memory	129
10. Interviewing	149
11. Executive functions	165
12. Slow processing	183
13. Reading and writing	195
Section Three: Unlocking dyslexic strengths	**216**
14. The truth about dyslexic strengths	219
15. Seeing the big picture	235
16. Understanding dyslexic strengths beyond big-picture thinking	249
17. Dyslexic strengths in real life	255
Final thoughts	262
Acknowledgements	264
References	265

Introduction

Dyslexia is a form of neurodivergence that affects an estimated one in 10 people – or around 700 million people worldwide. Yet despite this, once we leave school, it's hardly mentioned. Instead, we are left on our own to figure things out, often with very little support or understanding. This can make life very difficult.

Perhaps you've made it to higher education or the workplace, and suddenly you're expected to 'just manage', yet there are still endless tasks that feel overwhelming. For some, you may not yet have had a diagnosis and have no idea why certain tasks are so difficult. For others, you may have been given the label 'dyslexic' as an explanation for your challenges, but remain completely in the dark about the individual traits of dyslexia and any strengths associated with it. Even if you did have strategies that could help, years of struggling may have left your confidence in tatters, and the limiting emotions of fear, shame and anxiety can make it feel easier to stay quiet and suffer than speak up for what you need.

This is where this book comes in. Written by a dyslexic person, for dyslexic people, my aim is to help you understand dyslexia better so that you can move forwards with greater confidence and a toolkit of strategies to help you in day-to-day life. I'm not going to pretend there is a simple fix that will take your dyslexia away, but there are strategies that make challenges easier, that rebuild confidence and help you unlock your dyslexic strengths. Most importantly, this book will help you realise you are not alone in this challenge and create a manual for success.

To do this effectively, I have broken the book down into clear, accessible sections:

Introduction

The first section is the introduction, which covers a few different topics. I begin with my own story, as someone who struggled daily in the workplace and grew tired of how little support there was for adults, and therefore decided to create change by starting a business dedicated to adult dyslexia.

I then take a quick look at what dyslexia actually is and how it can affect our lives.

The three areas that every dyslexic needs to focus on in order to achieve success are: 1) unlocking dyslexic confidence, 2) unlocking dyslexic strategies and 3) unlocking dyslexic strengths. These are explored in much greater detail as we move through each subsequent section of the book, in which I help you gain clarity on your current situation and provide tried-and-tested strategies to help you navigate each of the three important areas. Together, they form a framework that can be applied to any situation you face and will help you navigate challenges and ensure you are able to make the most of the value and opportunity that neurodiversity can bring.

Section 1: Unlocking dyslexic confidence

This section is the key to helping you understand, accept and move forwards with improved confidence as a dyslexic person. Without improving your confidence in yourself, your abilities and your right to advocate for what you need, it's very difficult to make any progress, so please do read this section.

Section 2: Unlocking dyslexic strategies

Now that you're feeling more confident – which is essential for success – it's time to look at what strategies are needed to manage dyslexic challenges. To do this, we need to understand how and why dyslexia affects our lives, from issues with memory, slow processing and executive function, to fatigue, burnout and problems getting – and keeping – a job. Often, many of us don't even realise how much dyslexia is impacting us.

We then take each challenge in turn, breaking down strategies and solutions that will help you navigate dyslexic challenges. As many of you know, it isn't just about knowing what strategies work. We also help you think about how to best implement these in your life so you can be more consistent.

Section 3: Unlocking dyslexic strengths

Dyslexia isn't just about challenges – it has lots of exciting and valuable strengths. However, when discussing these, many people use overly simplistic language and terms like 'gift' or 'superpower'. It can be hard to relate to these when you have spent so much time struggling. In this section, I will help you understand what dyslexic strengths really mean to you as an adult. It isn't just about explaining terms you have heard a hundred times before, but about helping you build a path to unlocking your potential by ensuring your dyslexic strengths are valued by everyone and feel reliable enough to be used every day.

So this book is for you, if you're . . .

- . . . tired of struggling along alone and want help managing your dyslexia
- . . . fed up with being patronised and fed glib messages that minimise your struggles
- . . . keen to learn more about the science of dyslexia in real-world terms
- . . . ready to do the work to help yourself

Read on – you're in the right place!

My dyslexic story

Every dyslexic person has a story, and I am no different. I wanted to start by sharing my experience of being dyslexic, as from school through to adult life, the reality of managing dyslexia has defined and shaped the approach that I am now sharing with you.

I was diagnosed with dyslexia at a young age, when I was seven, and with ADHD at 29. Having a dyslexia diagnosis this early makes me one of the 'lucky' ones, meaning that for much of my life I had some sense of why I was struggling and I was able to access support. Although I am so grateful for this, it certainly never felt easy.

My first memory of dyslexia and its impact is of having to switch schools. Teachers at my first school had started to realise when I was very young – before my diagnosis – that I was struggling more than expected with certain tasks; I was chatty and articulate when I was speaking but I couldn't translate those ideas into words on the page. In fact, at this point I couldn't write much beyond a poorly constructed sentence. It was the late 1990s and the school didn't see dyslexia as something worth providing support for. However, I was struggling, I urgently needed help, and my mum has always said that from a young age it was obvious I was capable but the school was failing me. So, she made a decisive choice and ripped me out of my school mid-term and sent me to a new one that provided dyslexic support, to ensure I did not fall further behind.

The impact of my dyslexia didn't end once I'd moved to a more appropriate school: nearly every report or interaction involved a reminder that I needed to 'work harder' or that I was a 'bright kid' that just needed help accessing that. Some teachers even went as far as to repeatedly try to remove me from their classrooms so they wouldn't have to deal with my additional needs. As a defence mechanism, when I was a teenager I started lying to my friends, telling them that I had hardly tried and that was why I hadn't got a good grade, when in reality I had spent hours trying but still hadn't done well.

All of these small moments of struggle profoundly impacted the way I felt about myself, chipping away at my confidence and self-belief. Every day felt like a battle with my brain, and by the time exams came around my grades, although good, felt to me like they came rubber stamped with: 'not able to fulfil potential'. I was the classic dyslexic who had great ideas but couldn't get them down on paper. It felt like a curse and all I wanted was to rip out my brain and get a new one.

The support I got at school felt like the bare minimum, but for many pupils today, it would be a huge step up from what is currently provided. Even so, what truly changed the game was the fact that my mum worked tirelessly with me and believed I deserved dyslexic support – and made sure I got it. My parents also refused to accept my negative outlook and constantly reinforced that I wasn't defined by my challenges, but that they were simply a sign we needed to find a different approach. I couldn't hear it at the time, but it is exactly this ethos that later sparked my desire to start my company, Dyslexia in Adults.

I muddled along and made it through school and university, thankfully with extra time in my exams. At this point, I had a handful of strategies that my mum and I had built, which relied on my working significantly harder than others. This felt just about sustainable at university due to the free time I had, but was not a winning formula once I left.

It was now time to enter the world of work and figure out my next steps. I remember all my friends applying for grad schemes, but I didn't want to, for fear of not being able to pass the tests or my brain not fitting in at the high-paying companies that everyone around me was applying to. I felt like even if I could get through the door, the reality of my dyslexic challenges meant they wouldn't want 'someone like me'. The truth is that I was too scared to even try. Failure seemed inevitable due to my dyslexia, and that felt like going through exams all over again.

While I was doing my degree, I had thought about career paths. I was studying politics and was keen to follow my passion and felt excited to discuss ideas and build policies to help people, but when I started to consider how my dyslexia would impact me, I remembered all the articles I'd read about 'lazy' ministers who couldn't keep up with their work. In the articles, some ministers were judged for not doing their 'red boxes' (briefcases containing important documents that have to be read) after work hours and were therefore deemed not up to the task. That led to another big red cross mark over another career, as before I built coping strategies I often experienced extreme brain fog or exhaustion by the afternoon, which made me think it would not be possible for me to work late in the evenings reading complex documents. What is gut-wrenching is that this wasn't just another career I wasn't willing to try for fear of being inadequate – this was closing the door on my dreams and passion.

The same was true for other potential careers. By the time I graduated from university I had a long list of jobs and roles that I had written off as things I was 'incapable of succeeding at' because they were incompatible with dyslexia. Conversely, there was nothing on my list of jobs I 'could have a go at'. I was afraid of showing the truth of how hard certain tasks were for me because I felt like employers would then decide I would be too much effort – much like my teachers did – and they would prefer someone 'normal' (whatever normal means).

I tried to think about what an 'easy' job could be, to help me get started and learn the world of work. This led to me accepting a data entry job. Thinking back now, I am not sure why I thought all those other careers would be 'impossible' and a data entry job would work for my dyslexic mind. But at the time, I didn't consider how dyslexia made easy tasks hard for me – I just thought if it was deemed 'easy', even I could do it. Of course, in reality, inputting hundreds of numbers a day was probably the worst job I could have chosen for my brain.

Not surprisingly, that job didn't go well, and I almost got fired multiple times. However, like my mum and teachers had always said, I was incredibly capable at other things. My non-verbal communication skills started to shine and I would notice problems and provide solutions that showed my ability to my bosses. They quickly moved me into roles that centred on building relationships, which felt like a glimmer of hope that maybe I had a chance of finding a career that worked for me.

It wasn't all plain sailing, though. During this period I was consistently told during my annual reviews that I needed to 'pay more attention to small errors', or else I had to have my probation extended because I couldn't get to grips with roles as quickly as they wanted. In despair, I would regularly look up dyslexia advice online, wondering why there was nothing specific for adults; often, all I'd find was a checklist of dyslexic struggles that fitted me but that provided few or no answers. If I was extra lucky I might find a story about a dyslexic person who had been successful, but all it would say was something along the lines of 'focus on your strengths'. I would think to myself, *HOW, THOUGH?!* I was confused about what my strengths actually were. These stories felt so frustrating because the central theme always seemed to be that they relied on having your own business or being so successful you could have a personal assistant to support your challenges. Neither scenario felt like advice I could use in my twenties in junior corporate roles. I felt fearful that I would be trapped in a constant cycle of glimmers of my value alongside the daily drudgery of hours of hard work only to be criticised for the same dyslexic challenges that had haunted me my entire life. I would always think to myself, *Someone should really focus on adult dyslexia; we spend billions supporting kids but adults need help, too.*

Years went by and I started working at a large tech company in London, where the usual cycle repeated itself: a job interview where potential employers witnessed my strong communication skills, then starting the job and experiencing the usual challenges setting in, resulting in my employers extending my probation and constantly picking up on dyslexic challenges. After one particular majorly embarrassing mistake I admitted everything was due to dyslexia. They knew I was dyslexic but, like most employers, they didn't understand what that meant and how broad the challenges were. In response, they asked, 'How can we help you?' but of course I had no idea. I had scraped through education with hard work and extra time in exams but no one had taught me how to handle being dyslexic as an adult. When I got home, I tried googling it again, only to find nothing aside from suggestions to use spellcheck. Again, I thought, *Someone should do something!*

At this point it had become a habit of mine to move jobs every few years (getting bored easily was a behavioural pattern that I didn't recognise until much later), convinced that a new job was the answer to my problems. This time, I decided to go to a fast-moving start-up, hoping that this might play to my dyslexic strengths rather than just trying to avoid things I found challenging. I felt like I had finally cracked the sense of career success and satisfaction other people were talking about when I made a suggestion that brought in a lot of new leads (I was in sales at the time, so this was a huge win). But as always, dyslexic challenges weren't far away and the following week my boss noticed a big mistake in one of the emails I had written to a prospective client, and screamed at me.

The combination of the jolt of that stressful moment, seeing how the careers of those around me had started to really take off, and being tired of what by my mid-twenties felt like a predictable pattern of struggles made me realise I couldn't go on like this. I knew from my experience at school and as a child that having the right dyslexic support made life easier and I knew that no one was providing it for adults. So, one evening in November 2019, on the way home, I opened my phone and started an Instagram account called Dyslexia in Adults.

There wasn't a plan – there was only desperation. I knew that I couldn't continue as I had been and that I had to make a change. I knew I had to figure this out or else the same cycle of mistakes and awkward conversations would recur. That I would ultimately lose out on a lot of potential income because I was building a career that was beset by endless setbacks – but more than that because I had no idea how to deal with any of the areas I found difficult. And, most importantly, my confidence was by now at such a low level it's a miracle I could attend an interview and convince anyone I was competent, because I certainly didn't believe I was.

I'm not sure why it surprised me, but it did: the account lit up in a few weeks and within a few months I had 5,000 followers. I received hundreds of comments and DMs from people telling me that they were dealing with the same problems I had shared and that they were just struggling along in silence exactly like I was. They had no idea what worked and also eye-rolled every time dyslexia was called a 'gift', when all they saw was constant mistakes and exhaustion.

Another few years ticked by, with me working at one of the biggest companies in the world while still running my Dyslexia in Adults account. During this time I began to notice how much I struggled with interrupting people, regulating my focus and getting started on tasks that felt boring. I thought I was starting to figure out the issues around my dyslexia by sharing problems and ideas with my community on Instagram, but after the hundredth tough conversation with my boss, I realised that something more than dyslexia was at play.

I was eventually asked to leave that job (with a settlement), being told the usual story I had heard my entire life – that 'I was clearly very smart but this job didn't seem to align with my skills'. It was through learning more about dyslexia and the specific challenges that this role had highlighted that I understood that something else must be wrong, because I felt like I was moving mountains every day just to do the basics. I finally clicked that I also have ADHD – which came with all the grief, anger and frustration that commonly accompany a neurodiversity diagnosis later in life.

I had started Dyslexia in Adults because I knew I couldn't continue how I was – exhausted, frustrated and afraid of 'failing' – for the rest of my life. But at a deeper level, I wanted to achieve a potential that I knew was there, deep down inside – skills that others had constantly commented on but which I didn't have the tools to access fully. I had so little confidence that I would constantly make jokes about how useless I was, but still there was a tiny voice in my head telling me that I could achieve something if I just knew how to handle my neurodiversity.

And so I educated myself and learned. I did this in several ways:

- Reading research papers and rooting out what little advice there is for adults.
- Reading what was available for children and thinking about how adults could use that same advice.
- Figuring things out for myself, based on learning about dyslexic challenges and trialling strategies to overcome them.
- Drawing on knowledge and tips from people in my Dyslexia in Adults community.
- Doing a qualification to improve my knowledge about executive function.
- Going to conferences and connecting with world-class speakers who would go on to present inside my monthly membership for dyslexics and give me invaluable advice.

Now that I have the answers for myself, I want to help you.

Since Dyslexia in Adults began, I have run online workshops with large companies, started a podcast and worked with thousands of people to help them realise that managing neurodiversity is possible and, dare I even add, easy? My message is that their strengths are real and valuable, but without using trite phrases like 'dyslexia is your superpower'.

And that is the message and purpose of this book, too: it's here to put the challenges dyslexic adults face in all areas of life at the centre of the conversation. But more than that, I want to help you realise that your brain isn't broken, it's just different. Different can be difficult, but there's no reason you can't achieve everything you have dreamed of. You don't have to shrink from anything – you just need to learn how to handle it differently. Inspiring quotes alone won't help you manage your dyslexia, but confidence, clarity and strategies around how to use your dyslexic strengths will.

So let's get into it!

1
Understanding dyslexia

> **Chapter summary**
>
> **Why this chapter is important**
>
> The goal of this book is to help you make sense of where you are now and to build a path to move forwards in your relationship with dyslexia. In order to do this, you need to know what dyslexia is, and isn't, and how it impacts everyday life.
>
> **What you will learn**
>
> - What dyslexia actually is
> - How it can show up for different people, and some common problems
> - How a lack of understanding can cause issues with self-confidence and prevent you seeking appropriate support
> - How to identify which challenges are due to your dyslexia
> - Busting some common myths about dyslexia

Dyslexia is wildly misunderstood. Despite being recognised as a condition since 1887, many people still know very little about it, meaning we find ourselves having to teach them the basics again and again. What's more, even some dyslexic people don't understand the true extent of what it means to live with dyslexia. I often say that dyslexia is viewed through a very narrow lens. For instance, if I tell you that I am dyslexic, chances are you won't picture a woman in her thirties; you're far more likely to imagine a five-year-old boy struggling to read. But those kids grow up – and although our struggles may evolve, our brains don't magically change when we turn 18.

To truly understand dyslexia, I want to start at the beginning. Dyslexia affects multiple areas of the brain involved in processing information – our brains work differently from those of people who don't have dyslexia. This can lead to a wide range of issues – but it also brings many positives. For example, a person who can't spell 'jewellery' can still be an invaluable member of a team at work and might make an amazing partner or parent!

It makes sense that, since dyslexia affects many areas of the brain, it has a significant impact on many areas of life. Deep down, you probably know that you're different from people without dyslexia in ways that go far beyond just reading and writing – but perhaps you worry about using dyslexia as a 'card' or excuse when you find other things difficult. The truth is you likely *do* find some other things harder than others do.

The good news is that understanding and accepting your brain – and how and why you do things – is one of the more effective ways to learn to manage dyslexia successfully.

How to think about adult dyslexia

As our lives evolve, so does our dyslexia. We may no longer be children struggling to learn to read and sound out words, but instead adults in meetings or court hearings or working in factories, feeling anxious about being asked to read aloud. We may no longer face spelling tests, yet still receive email replies pointing out our spelling mistakes.

The core challenges often remain the same – but the circumstances and situations in which they arise continue to evolve.

A lot of the experiences and impacts of dyslexia in adulthood stems from how it affected us as children. Currently, the majority of adults who are dyslexic were educated in systems that rarely recognised or supported the neurodivergence. This lack of early understanding can also have significant, lasting repercussions on how we manage our dyslexia today.

Here are some of the most common problems dyslexic adults face:

1. **Fear and confusion**
   There's no blueprint for adult dyslexia, and few people to help you answer simple but important questions – like whether you should tell your boss about your dyslexia, and what support you can reasonably expect. This can all heighten the anxiety you already feel.

2. **Exhaustion**
   Many people aren't actively managing their dyslexia – they're learning to hide the differences it creates by working harder. This often leads to burnout and long hours spent trying to minimise the effects that others might notice.

3. **Unique ideas are undervalued**
   There is no doubt that dyslexic thinking holds great value and power (more on this in section 3), but difficulties with breaking down ideas or a lack of confidence can mean those ideas aren't shared.

4. **Problems with executive function**
   As children, you may have had support systems in place to help with organisation and planning (known as executive functions). But in adulthood, the responsibility for managing your life becomes much harder. It's not that these challenges didn't exist in childhood, but the safety nets disappear when you're an adult, and the consequences are much greater.

5. **Working memory issues**

   This important but not well-understood element of dyslexia is often at the root of many challenges. It is your brain's post-it note, holding information for short periods of time. It creates difficulties in remembering key details, organising your thoughts and constantly losing items.

6. **Confidence gets shredded**

   By far the biggest challenge I see for adults with dyslexia is the impact it has on confidence. Years of small mistakes or difficulties accumulate, painting a picture in your mind that you're 'useless' or a 'burden', simply because you're different. You struggle to see the value in your strengths because you're constantly having to work hard to overcome the challenges. And just to be clear – I'm not saying I was any better, in case you feel judged.

Dyslexia is like a mojito

Dyslexia shows up differently for different people. To explain my thinking and lighten the mood, I like to think of it as a very special cocktail...

Have you ever had a mojito made exactly the same way twice? I doubt it: no bartender makes it identically. You broadly know what you're getting when you order the cocktail – rum, sugar and mint – but the specifics of how it's put together can vary significantly. Let's just talk about the rum, for starters: dark rum, spiced rum, and then there is the quantity. I am confident that the amount of rum carefully measured at a fancy London cocktail bar will differ greatly from a local joint in Havana, where the pour might blow your socks off! Clearly, then, the same ingredients can concoct very different outcomes.

Dyslexia is no different. The struggles each person faces reflects the unique, heady cocktail of how their brain works, their prior experiences, and their own acceptance of and attitude towards their dyslexia. It makes for an interesting mix!

Is it me, or is it dyslexia?

Something that I see repeatedly is people not knowing how to differentiate between challenges caused by their dyslexia and those stemming from other factors. This is partly because many of the classic dyslexic symptoms are still poorly understood, so it's easy to assume that the problems you're experiencing are a 'you' problem, rather than part of the broader picture of dyslexia. This can be problematic, for a number of reasons:

1. **Lack of understanding is a vacuum for self-loathing**
   I knew dyslexia affected my ability to spell and read words, and I understood there were a lot of challenges that made me feel like I wasn't 'normal'. But what dyslexia exactly meant – beyond the simplistic explanation – was confusing. This matters not just because understanding your dyslexia is important, but because the absence of that understanding leaves a vacuum. And in that vacuum, it's easy to believe you're stupid. You're not.

   Understanding dyslexia is one of the most important steps in building effective strategies. To manage dyslexia successfully, you have to do it *proactively*. Yet, time and time again, you don't realise how dyslexia is affecting you until it's too late – until that moment of 'uh oh, I'm struggling more than I should' hits. Only then do you start to wonder if dyslexia might be the cause.

   But when you understand your brain and the challenges that shape your experience, you can make proactive decisions *before* things go wrong. This not only makes dyslexia easier to manage, but taking decisive action and asking for help is often far better received than seeking support only after you've made a mistake. All of this helps you feel better about yourself and your actions, too, and feeds into your confidence going forwards.

2. **People may question and invalidate your experience**
   Some people – perhaps out of kindness – may say things like, 'Oh, everyone struggles with that.' They may be trying to make you

feel better, but it can be deeply invalidating. The truth is, many of the challenges I've shared throughout this book are experienced by people with and without dyslexia. What makes it dyslexia is the *depth* of those experiences and the *consistency* with which they've shown up throughout your life. Try not to let other people make you doubt yourself; you know where your struggles lie, and their true impact on all facets of your life.

3. **It can be hard to pinpoint which challenges are linked to dyslexia**
   Most of my clients come to me knowing something isn't working. They've usually faced significant challenges and often relate strongly to my story. But unpicking exactly what's going on – and identifying which challenges are linked to dyslexia – can be difficult. To start with, I ask them to reflect across the week and answer two questions:

   I. What makes you feel so exhausted you wish you could leave work immediately?
   II. What makes you feel so much dread you would rather pull a sicky than do it?

These strong feelings are often signs that your brain is being asked to do things that don't come naturally. And that's where we can start to explore how dyslexia may be at play and work out how to progress.

The wild dyslexic myths

Unfortunately, there are still a lot of myths and misconceptions about dyslexia. These are not only wrong – they're ultimately harmful. They distort how people perceive our challenges and prevent them from seeing what we are capable of with the right support. They also create barriers in employment and education.

Here are some of the more common ones:

1. 'People with dyslexia aren't smart or capable enough to do degrees or hold down jobs.'

Some people are shocked when they learn what dyslexic individuals have achieved. They wrongly believe that being dyslexic affects intelligence or capacity to achieve in life. Common reactions include:

- Surprise that you got into university or another higher education setting – let alone completed it.
- Amazement that you read books.
- Confusion that dyslexic people can be successful in their careers.

2. 'Dyslexia is "worse" for those who speak English.'

Although I do wish the English language would cut me some slack occasionally and start spelling things phonetically, it's not the language that makes me dyslexic – it's my brain's processing. The vagaries of the English language just add stress.

I've spent three years learning Spanish, and I still can't spell in it, despite it being considered easier for dyslexic learners.

3. 'Dyslexia is for stupid rich kids.'

I remember being told that dyslexia was just a label middle-class families used for their 'thick' kids, and that it doesn't exist. I think this incorrect view might have fallen out of favour slightly, which I am grateful for, but it was so common when I was younger that my grandfather didn't want people to know I was dyslexic because he feared it would mean they would think I was thick.

4. 'Dyslexia can be prayed away.'

In some cultures, people take dyslexic children to church to try to 'pray it away'. This, of course, only increases the sense of shame – the opposite of what helps dyslexic people reach their potential.

5. 'Coloured sheets help dyslexics read.'

One of the common interventions for dyslexic people is to use coloured sheets to stop text moving on a page. However, this is actually a separate issue called Irlen Syndrome – which some dyslexic people do have, but not all.

2
Dyslexic traits

> **Chapter summary**
>
> **Why this chapter is important**
>
> Although dyslexia affects everyone differently, there are some traits that commonly occur. These are often oversimplified to 'problems with reading and writing', but this misses the nuance, and how they affect us in adulthood. In this chapter, I go through them one by one, exploring the different aspects and bringing them to life with stories.
>
> **What you will learn**
>
> - What dyslexic traits are and how they impact everyday life, with specific examples for: reading, writing, processing speed, executive function and other impacts of dyslexia.
> - What dyslexic strengths you might have.
> - Co-occurrence of dyslexia and other neurodiversity, and the traits of those other forms of neurodiversity.

Many of us recognise some dyslexic traits, but we often underestimate their full impact and don't appreciate how they show up in adulthood. Yet gaining a deeper understanding is the key to learning how to work with dyslexia and unlock its potential. The guide below therefore explores some of the core traits and how they can affect day-to-day life.

The examples I've shared are here both to help you have a laugh and to remind you that you're not alone in having these experiences – millions of people face the same challenges. This is important, because feeling alone and like you're the problem often results in confidence being crushed and prevents you from using strategies effectively.

It's also important to understand that dyslexia isn't simply about 'can' or 'can't' – it's about how much *effort* it takes to complete a task.

So, let's get into it.

Reading

Reading is, of course, one of the most commonly recognised dyslexic challenges, but here I want to break down all the ways it impacts us as adults.

Difficulties processing information

For many, adult reading difficulties aren't so much about being able to break down the sounds in a word, but about processing and truly understanding the overall concepts. This can cause all sorts of problems, such as:

1. Finding reading incredibly tiring.
2. Difficulty fully digesting complex documents.
3. Needing complete focus to be able to read.
4. Fear of reading aloud.

Here are a few examples that I am sure you will relate to.

1. Pushing on a door that says 'pull'

I can't tell you how many times I've had to fib to people that I didn't see the 'push' or 'pull' sign when I'm feeling caught out fumbling with a door longer than is considered 'normal'. You know the times I mean – when you've clearly read that it says 'pull' but continue to push anyway. Then, seconds later (which always feel like minutes in situations like this), you realise what the sign actually says – and feel like a total idiot.

2. Misreading flight gate numbers or train station names

Is there anything more nerve-wracking for a dyslexic than travelling? The cost of making a mistake is high, and the number of opportunities for error even higher. I've ended up at the wrong gate at airports many times, or, worse, confidently led other people the wrong way.

Recently, a good friend of mine – who is just as dyslexic as me – and I ended up at completely the wrong terminal in Naples due to misreading the signs repeatedly. Thankfully, both of us were fit enough to sprint across the airport at short notice and make our flight.

A woman from our weekly Dyslexia in Adults newsletter was not so lucky when a similar thing happened to her on the London Underground. She got so lost and confused that she wasn't able to process the writing on the signs and ended up being an hour late for a first date.

3. Booking tickets incorrectly

Train tickets, theatre tickets, plane tickets . . . they're always anxiety-inducing until you're in the venue or on the transport and confident nothing's gone wrong. Whenever I share examples of my own mishaps, I always get flooded with stories from others who have done the same.

For example, on my 30th birthday I paid for accommodation so that five of my friends could join me in Lisbon. They all paid for their flights – expensive in the height of summer – only for me to book an

Airbnb for one night, not two... I remember thinking at the time the accommodation was oddly cheap compared to the others I'd looked at!

These types of mistakes are mortifying, especially in front of other people; I am always grateful when they happen in private.

4. Reading a message and thinking it says something completely different

I've read countless messages – simple or complex – and thought that I have understood and replied to them perfectly, only to reread them the next day and realise my reply made no sense. Once, my friend asked about my vitamin D levels. It was 10 February, so I replied by telling him about my Valentine's Day plans... How on earth did my brain get that confused?

5. Finding it difficult to read a menu

Going out for a meal is meant to be a pleasurable experience, but for us dyslexics, it can create a lot of stress. Faced with a menu that might contain all sorts of unfamiliar words, we can freeze and panic and end up ordering something we don't actually want.

Of course the best way to avoid this is to look up the menu online first, so you can read it at your own pace and go to the meal knowing what you want, but this isn't always an option. And then there's deciphering handwriting on those blackboards that list the specials...

6. Reading, and following, recipes

Recipes pose some of the same challenges as menus. However, it's very easy for us to misread 'tsp' and 'tbsp' and add too much or too little of some vital ingredient. We might also misread the label on a jar and add the wrong ingredient altogether!

7. Not being able to read for pleasure

It follows, then, that reading isn't always pleasurable for us. I've always looked so fondly at people who can curl up with a good book or read before bed to wind down (hello, racing thoughts from ADHD!). I admire those who can talk about the latest book that broadened their horizons or boast about how many books they have read that year or how quickly they've raced through the latest must-read title.

My reality with reading is that I've probably read around 30 books in my life – if not fewer. For some of you that will seem like an impressive feat, but I promise I struggled through every last one of them. Not so much because of the words themselves, but because of the energy it takes to read properly. There are therefore only limited times in my life when I've had the capacity to read for pleasure.

8. Immediately thinking 'no' to long text

Clients often tell me they open a long email or an overwhelming message and their brain's response is immediate: *Nope. Declined. No thank you.* This is because they know exactly how much effort it will take to process it. This can obviously cause issues, whether you're at work or having to read a long document when buying a house or dealing with medical correspondence.

Real-world story

Tijuana is a place in Mexico I've heard of, but the first time I saw it written down, I had no idea how to pronounce it. I was 21, in my first job, frightened every day by the reality of my dyslexia. I'd just had a mini promotion and was in a meeting, looking at a map. I tried to sound out 'Tijuana' as best I could, but didn't realise it was the place I had heard of. I messed it up, and everyone in the meeting fell about laughing at what felt like such a stupid mistake.

For most people, this would have been a bit embarrassing but not the end of the world. For me, I remember distinctly crying in the toilets wishing so desperately that my brain worked differently. I promised myself I would never speak up in a meeting again (even though that was a ridiculous thing to think). I wish I could go back in time and let that girl know what I have achieved since then.

9. Anxiety about presenting

Many of my clients share with me their anxiety around presenting, particularly with PowerPoint slides they haven't seen before. Reading the slides directly and processing in real time what is being said often feels impossible. Instead, they need to practise over and over and OVER again to memorise every detail, because using the slides as prompts can feel too scary or difficult.

> **Real-world story**
>
> Recently, my oldest friend got married and kindly asked me to do a reading. I was so touched and honoured – not just because it meant being part of her wedding, but because she believed I wouldn't mess it up.
>
> I'm pleased to say I read it beautifully, not stuttering once over a very complex poem (she could've cut me some slack!). But in true dyslexic fashion, I had practised it to death. My poor mum, who was also going to the wedding, had to hear it over and over – she must have been sick of me, and the poem, by the time I read it at the wedding.

Writing

Everything about dyslexia is more complex than I wish it were, and writing is no different. It's likely that at some point when you've mentioned dyslexia at work or another setting, your manager has replied, 'No problem, we have spellcheck.' If only it were that simple. The following are some examples of the difficulties we may face when it comes to writing:

1. Getting your ideas down

Dyslexia is often described as 'difficulty getting your ideas down on paper' – a challenge that's haunted me my whole life. As I said earlier, it's not as simple as 'can' or 'can't'. It's about the gap between what's in your head and what you manage to get out into the world. This can result in writing and rewriting endlessly and still feeling like it wasn't good enough.

> **Real-world story**
>
> My client told me that when she broke up with her boyfriend, she was so worried she wouldn't be able to articulate her thoughts properly she decided to write everything out, film herself saying it and watch it back – to make sure her words were clear. This is a perfect example of how it's not about ability, but about the effort required to reach the outcome we want.

Procrastinating

Sometimes, the challenge of breaking down ideas and expressing our thoughts can feel like climbing Everest – so daunting that you don't want to start or you convince yourself it's not worth even trying. This leads to procrastination, which wastes time and can lead you to miss deadlines.

Confusing sentences

Working through the challenges of phonological processing, working memory and organising thoughts simultaneously can make sentence structure and grammar – never automatic to begin with – fall off a cliff. The result? Sentences that are poorly structured or confusing.

I often find that when I write something, it makes perfect sense when I read it aloud before hitting send. But when I revisit the email, I cringe and feel that a four-year-old would sound more eloquent than me.

Real-world story

Recently, my boyfriend read over my shoulder as I drafted an important message. I had asked him to do this: I needed him to review it, to make sure it conveyed my point clearly. I've long stopped caring about what friends and family think about spelling mistakes in messages, but this one was going to someone else.

My boyfriend made significant changes to the sentence structure and later, very kindly and gently, told me: 'Sometimes your texts take me a second to decipher.'

I won't change or take more care over non-important messages – because it requires too much energy to reach such a high bar, especially for someone you message frequently – but knowing that he was a bit confused by every message I sent did make me wince a little.

Real-world story

Despite all the issues I had at school, I chose a humanities subject at university – which meant writing a lot of essays. The feedback I always got from tutors was that my sentences were 'flabby'. My dissertation felt like a huge task, involving writing 12,000 words. My first draft prompted my tutor, again with every kindness, to say: 'Natalie, you have great ideas, but the sentences are a little flabby. You need to make sure you double-check your writing.' If only he knew how many times I had already read over it. My mum and dad ended up reading it late into the night a few days before submission, sending me detailed tracked changes.

2. Spelling challenges

I have always maintained that if dyslexia were just about difficulties with reading and spelling, I wouldn't mind as much – but the truth is, the challenges are much broader and more complex. That doesn't make these common frustrations with writing any easier, though:

Spelling and homophones

People sometimes say you're 'more dyslexic' in certain languages, which is obviously ridiculous. But English does have its traps – like homophones: words that sound the same but are spelled differently. For instance:

> there v their
> which v witch
> father v farther
> break v brake

The frustrating part of this problem is that spellcheck often misses these mistakes, because technically they are correct words. Of course, there are other tools available – many dyslexics use Grammarly, for instance, which helps significantly.

We also commonly transpose letters in words that contain the same letters, such as 'angle' and 'angel' or 'dairy' and 'diary'.

> ### Real-world story
>
> My favourite story is when I tried to explain dyslexia to a boyfriend and told him I had a 'weird Brian' instead of a 'weird brain'. Thankfully, I think that example conveyed my point about transposing letters nicely. But for months afterwards, every mistake was met with a comment about my 'weird Brian', which the boyfriend found funny but I found embarrassing – and I didn't know how to tell him to stop.

Spelling simple words wrong

It's not just difficult words that dyslexics struggle with – it's often the simple ones that trip us up. This can be embarrassing if other people see your mistake, or frustrating if you have to reformat an entire sentence just to get your point across.

Examples of simple words that have recently tripped me up are: orange, growth and Saturday.

Complete confusion on spelling

Dyslexic people are commonly baffled by how a word is structured. This can be incredibly frustrating in lots of ways, though it's also a good way to help people understand the difference between dyslexia and general spelling difficulty. For example, dyslexics may feel totally lost on where to even begin spelling confusing words such as 'occasion', whereas someone with mild spelling issues might just wonder if it has two Cs.

> ### Real-world story
>
> One thing I often laugh about with my coaching clients is the weird words shops and venues use for their Wi-Fi passwords. Why do they have to make them so hard to spell? Or maybe I just can't imagine what it would be like to find spelling easy . . .
>
> A recent one that floored me was 'croissant'. If I asked you to close your eyes right now and think about how to spell it, are you merely wondering if there are two Rs or are you totally flummoxed on where to begin? If you're in the latter camp, that's your dyslexia rearing its head.

Processing speed

Dyslexia can leave you feeling like it's easier to say you 'can't' do something rather than trying and then feeling embarrassed when you find it difficult. A big part of that stems from difficulties with processing speed.

That idea – that someone would limit themselves because they feel they 'can't' – is awful and needs to stop. Processing speed has nothing to do with how much you can learn or what amount of information you can process. It's about:

1. How information comes in.
2. What you need to understand it.

I won't deny that this is frustrating and often embarrassing. You can have something explained to you and still feel confused – then a few minutes later, it clicks. That delay might only be a couple of seconds, but it has repercussions. Even when you know the delay is due to issues with processing speed, it's easy to default to giving yourself hurtful labels, such as 'thick'. Also, when someone has explained something to you three times and you're still looking at them like they are speaking a foreign language, it's mortifying.

What's important to understand is that processing speed affects not just how long it takes you to grasp the basics, but how long it takes to build a deep, detailed understanding of the topic.

Dyslexics are able to really excel when we have the full picture. We explore this in detail in chapter 15.

Of course, many of us have sat in meetings and not understood what was going on, but slow processing speed shows up in lots of other areas of life, too. Here are just a few examples:

1. Talking to myself in the street

I am unashamed to admit that I often chat away to myself in public when I'm deep in thought. Usually, it's because I am replaying a story or conversation in my head, crafting the genius reply I wish I'd given. Sadly, this smart and witty response normally comes hours too late because I process things slowly, so I am left only able to win the argument in my daydreams. But don't worry – in those, I win every time!

2. Laughing late

Slower processing speed can mean you struggle to get a joke at the same time as everyone else. It can be hugely embarrassing when everyone is laughing and you start laughing five seconds later. You might learn to fake laugh, but then get caught out when the real laugh arrives – and people realise you didn't get it the first time.

3. Pretending to have hearing issues

I often tell people I have poor hearing, because sometimes it's easier than admitting I have slow processing. It just feels less embarrassing to laugh it off and joke about needing to get my ears cleaned out. In fact, many dyslexics actually do get their hearing tested because their partners think they're not listening, having been asked to repeat themselves so many times.

4. Having great ideas late in the day

When people haven't been taught how to process efficiently and to work with their dyslexia, they may start specific tasks without fully understanding what they're supposed to be doing. This means ideas and approaches to that task can arrive in the middle of a project, making it hard to begin and causing plans to shift throughout.

Many clients also tell me that they feel so embarassed when people ask, 'do you have any questions?' And it is only the next day that a flood of questions arrive.

Executive functions

Dyslexia can often come alongside a lot of issues with organisation, time management and task execution – these fall under the umbrella of 'executive functions'. Knowing what executive functions are and all the components that come under that banner is essential to fully understanding your dyslexia.

What are executive functions?

Think of them as your brain's CEO – the control centre that helps you appear 'together' and function as the adult you're expected to be.

Everyone has executive functions, but for neurodiverse people, the biochemistry that connects and activates this area of the brain doesn't always link up cleanly.

In summary, executive functions help you:

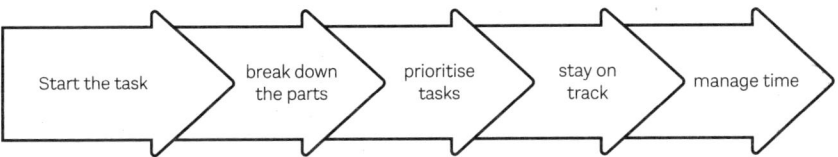

If you're nodding along in agreement, it's likely because a lot of the things that affect you as a dyslexic person – but that have little to do with reading or writing – are rooted in executive functions.

The 11 executive functions

1. Planning and prioritisation – figuring out what to do first.
2. Time management – understanding the passage of time.
3. Working memory – holding information in your head for short periods of time.
4. Organisation – organising concepts with ease and consistently.
5. Impulse control – not saying something you shouldn't or not thinking through your thoughts before speaking.

> 6. Task initiation – getting started on tasks in a timely manner.
> 7. Metacognition – evaluating and reflecting on your situation or actions.
> 8. Emotional control – staying regulated and calm.
> 9. Flexible thinking – being adaptable or changing your thinking.
> 10. Sustained attention – focusing on only one task at a time.
> 11. Goal-directed persistence – sticking with long-term goals.

Why your dyslexia gets worse when you're tired

Executive functions go offline or work less effectively when you're tired, stressed or hungry. So if you feel like your dyslexia (or other neurodivergence) gets worse under these conditions, you aren't going mad – it's science!

Working memory and why you must understand it

Working memory is like a mental Post-it note. It temporarily stores incoming information until your brain decides what to do with it – such as transferring it to long-term memory or ditching it.

Its capacity and duration are limited for everyone, but for neurodiverse people, it's even more restricted. Working memory affects both your ability to retain key details for a short period of time, and to organise and plan your thoughts. Therefore, it's often the root of many dyslexic challenges. For this reason, we explore it in detail – along with strategies to support it – in chapter 9.

Forgetting key details

One of the most consistent frustrations I hear from clients is forgetting small but important details – this can be someone's name or the date of their anniversary or an important work task that someone mentioned in passing. Commonly, it leaves you with an exhausting, constant sense that you have forgotten something. Over time, this can really impact your perception of yourself and create a feeling of uselessness, especially when these slip-ups happen repeatedly.

> ### Real-world story
>
> I have struggled with working memory issues on countless occasions, but one incident in particular stands out. A few years ago, I was in a cafe that had shared toilets within a larger complex. To access them, you needed a code. When I asked where the toilet was, the staff gave me complex instructions about its location, and a four-digit code. My working memory had to hold both sets of information, all while my stress levels were rising, which reduced my capacity further. Nightmare! This is how it went...
>
> The first time I went back to the counter it was to check if the toilets were to the left or the right.
>
> The second time was because I couldn't find the loo.
>
> The third time was when I realised I had forgotten the code.
>
> The fourth time I tried, I was so busy repeating the code aloud – '7435, 7435, 7435' – that I wasn't focusing and tripped and cut my knee.
>
> I haven't been back to the cafe since.

Other impacts of dyslexia

Dyslexia is about how your brain works. It's not just about reading and spelling – it's a lot of things. (I know I'm repeating this message, but that's because it's important!) Don't underestimate its impact or how far-reaching this can be.

Left and right confusion

Many dyslexic people struggle with left and right. You might know which is which, yet in that split second you're asked, you struggle. This is something that can come up a lot in driving. I've even heard of people tattooing 'L' and 'R' on their hands because the usual trick – holding up an L-shape with your left hand – doesn't always work for us due to spatial processing issues.

Difficulties learning to drive

Learning to drive, and driving itself, is overwhelming. There are so many individual details to track. To help with the left and right confusion mentioned above, many dyslexic people prefer to say, 'driver's side' or 'my side' rather than 'left' or 'right', and/or use hand gestures to accompany verbal directions.

A lot of dyslexics also struggle with both the practical and the theory tests. For example, my dyslexic ex-boyfriend took the theory test eight times before finally passing his practical.

I still haven't learned to drive. This is partly because I've always lived in cities and haven't needed to, but also because when I was younger, my parents had a lot of anxiety about me driving and it made me feel like I 'can't' – even though I know I could if I tried. Somehow, though, I seem to always find a reason why it isn't possible.

Reasonable Adjustments

In the UK, the Driving and Vehicle Standards Agency offer something called 'Reasonable Adjustments' for people who are dyslexic (or have another form of neurodivergence).

> Reasonable Adjustments mean that you can take your driving instructor or the person who has accompanied you to the test with you as a passenger. In addition, the examiner should ask you what adjustments you need. These include how you prefer to be given directions, limiting directions to two at a time, and showing you a diagram before the independent driving section. To find out more, go to: https://www.bdadyslexia.org.uk/advice/adults/learning-to-drive

Struggling with detail

Dyslexic people can really struggle to notice small details. We've talked about how spotting spelling mistakes can feel impossible, but it's the same with numbers or small differences. These errors can cause people to make comments about us being lazy for not double-checking something, but that couldn't be further from the truth.

Mirroring issues

Dyslexia is well known for number and letter confusion – especially with b, d, p, q and a. Fonts designed for dyslexic readers often use weighted shapes to help distinguish these characters and make processing simpler.

Dyslexic strengths

Over the last few years, dyslexia has been increasingly recognised for its strengths – not just its challenges. For many in the community, this is a huge shift from how we've historically been treated. It's a real opportunity to be viewed as more than our difficulties.

Dyslexic strengths are often grouped into two core areas: 1) creativity and 2) the ability to see situations in a unique or unconventional way that allows for problems to be noticed and solved or for new ideas to be put forward.

We'll be exploring dyslexic strengths in more detail in section 3.

Co-occurrence of dyslexia and other neurodiversity

If you've been diagnosed with dyslexia, the likelihood of having another form of neurodiversity is quite high.

I'm always cautious with statistics here, as neurodiversity research is underfunded and underdeveloped, but the following figures are taken from reputable sources:

- Approximately 25–40 per cent of individuals with dyslexia also meet diagnostic criteria for ADHD.
- Around 40–50 per cent of children diagnosed with dyslexia show signs of dyscalculia.
- Estimates suggest that 30–50 per cent of people with dyslexia also experience motor coordination difficulties consistent with dyspraxia.
- Studies indicate that 5–10 per cent of individuals with autism spectrum disorder (ASD) also meet the criteria for dyslexia.

I was diagnosed with ADHD at the age of 29. One of the barriers to me truly accepting it was the feeling that I was 'too much' or somehow 'greedy' to have more than one neurodiversity, especially since I also have dyscalculia and dyspraxia (DCD). This, of course, is not true. What's more, it's really important to explore and consider the other forms of neurodiversity, because understanding your brain is essential to managing your neurodivergence successfully.

What are the other forms of neurodiversity?

Given that other forms of neurodiversity commonly co-occur with dyslexia, it makes sense to take a quick look at what they are:

ADHD

What it is: Difficulty regulating attention. You can't force yourself to focus when something is difficult or boring. The lack of dopamine makes doing rote tasks feel extremely difficult.

Examples:

- Needing more stimuli to focus – doing two things at once, which others misinterpret as distraction.
- Hyperfocus on things you enjoy, and zero focus on things you 'should do'.

Dyscalculia

What it is: Not just difficulty with mental arithmetic, but a confusion over the concept of numbers.

Examples:

- Difficulty estimating crowd sizes.
- Lack of understanding about percentages.

Dyspraxia (DCD)

What it is: A difficulty with processing spatial awareness, which can make you clumsy and struggle with everyday physical tasks.

Examples:

- Bumping into things or tripping up.
- Missing your mouth with food or drink.

- Stirring a pot and misjudging the space, so that food goes everywhere.
- Having trouble navigating crowds and traffic, whether on foot or in a vehicle.

Autism (ASD)

What it is: Autism presents across a broad spectrum and can cause many different challenges.

Examples:

- Differences in non-verbal communication style. Most notably understanding and utilising eye contact.
- Differences in social communication. Such as not valuing small talk or unspoken expectations.
- Detail oriented, valuing precise and specific instructions.
- Prefers routine and predictability, finding change difficult.
- Intense focus on specific topics or objects.
- Clear morals and values, with strong reactions to injustice.
- Sensitive to stimuli such as textures, sounds or smells.

Section One

Unlocking dyslexic confidence

Dyslexia can have a huge impact on your confidence, and when you have low confidence, many areas of life can become challenging. For this reason, the first of the three pillars for unlocking dyslexia is to help you build confidence in being dyslexic. In this section, we are going to break down exactly how to do that.

Our approach for achieving this is through having truthful conversations about managing dyslexia. This stems from the fact that the most consistent feedback I get from clients is: 'I can't believe I have never properly spoken about this before.' Many go on to tell me how therapeutic it feels to be honest about their experiences.

I believe that it's more than just cathartic: I believe that it's essential for driving success with dyslexia. By clearly seeing how you are managing dyslexia through hard work and masking, you are able to identify the pitfalls in this approach. You will begin to see that confidently leaning into the differences, rather than hiding behind them, is what actually works.

How to use this section

In this section we talk about the role of confidence and how the failures in the system for dyslexic people have moulded us. This can be a confronting but important read. Here is some advice on how to get the most out of this section:

- Have a cry. Be angry at how the system failed you. Acknowledge the truth of how much it has impacted you. Take all of those emotions and forge them into a determination to break the cycle – if not just for yourself, then for all the future dyslexics who might suffer.

- See the power in not being alone. It's no longer just you being frustrated: it's millions of others who have gone through exactly the same experiences. In this way, you can step out of your comfort zone and demand the support that you deserve. I have often noticed that when someone feels that their challenges with dyslexia are a personal failing, it can make dyslexia much harder to manage. This might look like feeling personally responsible for keeping up or that they are not good enough, which can lead to them staying small and struggling in silence. Realising that the problem is the system, not you, helps put an end to this situation.

- 'Growing my confidence' is a goal that many of us have, especially if we are aware of some of the ways dyslexia has impacted us. This section gives you a simple blueprint for *how* to create that shift and move forwards:
    - The first step in this journey, in chapter 3, is really seeing your dyslexia and its impacts, so you can identify the areas you need to change.
    - The next stage, in chapter 4, is changing your mindset about your dyslexia (even if that feels airy-fairy) so that you can grow in confidence.

- The final stage, in chapter 5, is taking practical and specific steps to protect and maintain your confidence. Don't skip any of these chapters, as each one has a role to play in fostering the real and significant change that you deserve.

3

Understanding why dyslexia impacts confidence

> **Chapter summary**
>
> **Why this chapter is important**
>
> Being dyslexic is hard work. Whether you realise it or not, years of accumulated struggles will have taken their toll and affected your self-belief. This chapter examines how and why being dyslexic is challenging, and some common tendencies and behaviours that develop as a result.
>
> **What you will learn**
>
> - The three key realities for dyslexics: 1) you've felt different from an early age, 2) cruel comments confirm our worst fears, and 3) dyslexic strengths don't feel like they're enough.
> - What the common dyslexic cycles are.
> - How to break each of those cycles.

Unlocking dyslexia is about more than just strategies: it's about learning to accept, and own, being different. Often, it's not just the challenges of dyslexia that are holding us back but our negative perception of ourselves – a perception that has been built up through thousands of micro-mistakes, frustrations and the constant comments to 'try harder', 'focus on double-checking your work' and 'try again'.

The reality of life with dyslexia

In this section we are going to unpack the impact that these frustrations and constant criticisms have had on us. The goal here is to hold up a mirror and really understand how dyslexia manifests. It's hard but important work, which will first help us recognise the extent to which your current system isn't working, before we then build the pattern that *does* work.

I've broken down this process into three key realities for dyslexics, which we'll examine in turn.

1. You've felt different from an early age

Being different in any capacity can be really difficult. This is as true for dyslexia as it is for any other type of difference. With dyslexia, the feeling of being different often starts young – while we are developing our sense of self – and deeply impacts how we perceive ourselves. This can erode confidence. Every day, you might experience little moments when you look at your peers and feel less capable than them. In school, you likely spent years sitting in classrooms not learning as quickly as other kids, or spending much longer on your homework only to get the same or even lower grades than your classmates. All of these things leave you feeling like you're different, in a bad way.

Many dyslexics never want people to know the extent to which they are struggling. It will perhaps only be the people closest to you who will have had a glimpse at the reality. In adult life, it's generally easier to mask the truth. To say you have bad hearing when you need more processing time, or to say something 'didn't take too long' when you spent all weekend working extra hours to scour for every spelling mistake. Your past experiences have taught you that it's best to hide the truth.

And the truth is that you are judging yourself against a standard that isn't achievable because your brain doesn't work in the same way as someone without dyslexia. It sounds obvious, but it's worth repeating.

You are striving to reach other people's 'normal' without any of the 'normal' tools.

This is made all the more frustrating because for most of us at school there was no support, or no meaningful support. Our only option was to work hard and hope that something clicked. In reality, for many, that meant we stayed quiet and tried to mask our challenges. It is these traits, learned out of necessity, that are the low-confidence habits we are now trying to change.

Real-world story

My teachers liked me and spoke kindly to me, but the truth is they didn't want me in their classes, and I knew it. This left me feeling like no one wanted the dyslexic kid – I was too much effort and normal was just easier. I often tell this story with a big laugh and a smile on my face, making people think it's funny, but in truth it's an experience that has had a long-lasting, damaging impact. Like most dyslexic people, I use humour to mask the truth of how much it bothered me.

Towards the end of my time at school, we chose our subjects by having an open day and discussing with teachers what subjects would be a good fit. For me, the answer was: none. No one wanted the dyslexic kid in their classroom. No one wanted to deal with my brain.

Here is how every conversation went:

'Natalie, [insert concerned face] you are such a smart kid.

'But . . .

'This subject isn't for you . . .

'It involves too much writing . . . [or insert any other classic dyslexic challenge]

'You would be better off doing . . . [any other subject]'

Room after room, teacher after teacher – they all said the same. The history department said history involved too much reading and that I should try science. The science department said spelling the scientific words would be too difficult and I should try maths. The maths department knew I had dyscalculia and was confused as to why I was even there.

Why?! Because the last thing they wanted to do was teach me. They knew I had to make an extra effort to learn and, even with that extra effort, I often didn't get the grades that were expected by the teachers. They didn't want what they felt was a weak link in their classrooms, reflecting badly on them.

It is hard to truly explain what this felt like, knowing deep down that my teachers didn't want to help me, didn't see the effort as worth it. Inevitably, this enforced my view that I was a burden. They didn't have to tell me: I knew.

Sadly, this happened twice, each time we had to choose our subjects. The second time was even worse, since I knew that the teacher felt that the previous two years of teaching me hadn't been worth the effort.

This really impacted me and lingered long into my career. I felt like no one would want to help me – that I and my dyslexia were something that people put up with but wished they didn't have to. The result was that it became very clear to me that I had to hide my issues, hoping that no one would realise the depth of them, otherwise they would reject me.

2. Cruel comments confirm our worst fears

When you are dyslexic, the mistakes and frustrations you have tried to keep to yourself will eventually be noticed by others, and they may put you down in such a hurtful or cruel way that their comments can form part of your image of yourself. Those comments can be the worst fear that we carry around – waiting and worrying that it will happen again – pushing us to mask our challenges even more.

Sadly, most dyslexics will have a story of when a challenge has resulted in an embarrassing or significant mistake. Sometimes people brush it off as a 'one-time' occurrence, but for many there will have been a time when we were let go from a job, told we were incapable, or heard something so hurtful that it stays with us for life.

These situations can commonly push dyslexic people to 'prove' to the world we aren't as incapable as others claimed, which can lead to great achievements. However, under the surface, the negative comments can severely damage confidence, which in turn can have significant impacts across our lives.

For many, that moment when someone cut you down with horrible words or let you go from a job can feel like the moment when you were 'seen' – they said what you have feared all along. That fear can make people afraid to share that they're dyslexic while simultaneously fearing that people will notice the slips of the mask that inevitably occur over time or when under pressure.

Being dyslexic isn't just about the internal feeling of knowing you aren't able to express your thoughts fully – it's also dealing with the external reality of being called 'stupid' or 'lazy', which is the very thing that we aren't.

The weight of others' opinions can hurt you deeply, because often we know we are capable of more.

It is also made so much more frustrating by the fact that most people have a limited understanding of dyslexia. They often don't realise that it manifests as much more than spelling challenges and therefore don't understand the wider problems we face. That means that when we have dyslexic challenges, many people will just think we're incapable, or whatever more hurtful insult they decide to use.

That level of judgement and criticism, even when you know you're dyslexic, can become internalised and leave you questioning yourself.

What if I am just stupid?

What if it isn't dyslexia?

What if I am just slow?

And it's this self-doubt that is the real issue – one that stops us from achieving our true potential. This is not about searching for external validation or striving for a good job for the sake of it. It is about showing the world we are more than our challenges.

Real-world story

When I was in the final years of school, I had a teacher whom I idolised. She taught my favourite subject, which I was planning on studying at university. I worked the hardest in this class, putting extra effort into my homework and trying to showcase what I was capable of.

One day, I went to speak to her about which university I should choose. I had already done some work on this and had set what I felt were realistic expectations and a few stretch goals if my hard work paid off. Without a second's thought, she said, '*You want to go to university? YOU?!*'

Her incredulous response spoke volumes about what she thought of me and my abilities: 'You're already struggling with your schoolwork. How could you ever keep up with the demands of university?!'

Coming from the person whom I had worked so hard to impress, this was devastating. Without hesitation, she had told me that she didn't think I was worthy of university. I'll never forget the red-hot feeling in my cheeks, wanting the ground to swallow me up.

At first that comment pushed me to work harder, to prove to myself and to her that her opinion of me was wrong. I pushed it aside, going to university, studying an essay subject (politics) and getting a 2:1, showing that it *was* possible – that I wasn't as useless as she had made out.

The reality was, though, that the comment had stayed with me. I would often think about it when writing essays or when I had to work harder than others. It made me feel like I wasn't capable enough to go to university and I was lucky I had got this far. That it was highly possible I would be 'found out' at any moment. It was a comment that felt like the truth of me and who I was, and that all the success and achievements could be pulled from me at any moment.

3. Dyslexic strengths don't feel like they're enough

At school, it's pretty obvious when you're behind and others are able to learn faster than you or get better results with less effort. Then once you start working, those fears and concerns you built up around being different make you worry that your challenges will be 'found out' and you'll be deemed not good enough. Again.

The feeling of being different doesn't end when we become adults. It just changes. Instead of noticing how quickly other people are doing maths problems, you see how capable people are at sending emails (and never forgetting the attachments).

Dyslexia brings with it many strengths and although you may know that and recognise the value of your ideas, it may feel like the world of work doesn't value them. That employers only want 'the basics done right': ensuring that there is never a spelling mistake, that emails are answered quickly or that presentations are perfect.

As dyslexics we have ideas about how teams should run, how processes can be improved, or how innovations can revolutionise businesses. These ideas can often feel like flukes that occur once in a while and don't feel consistent enough to build a career around. So when these ideas land, we are often not senior enough to be heard.

It can feel so confusing trying to navigate the reality of both having these flashes of brilliance and of simple tasks taking a long time or containing multiple mistakes. It can trigger self-doubt. You might start to wonder, *If I can't get the easy tasks right, what does that say about me? Am I worthy of doing this job?*

The biggest challenge for me was just figuring out how to be different in the workplace. I never knew what to say. Even when I was asking colleagues to check my work, I always felt like such a burden and found myself wishing and willing my brain to be better and more capable in those moments. I didn't care about the things I was good at because all I wanted was to be 'normal'.

Real-world story

Rude comments don't stop at school, despite being told over and over again that 'once you leave school, you'll be fine' or 'technology means that dyslexia isn't really a problem any more'. The truth is, yes, I am so glad that I'm no longer in education. But it's not like my brain is now coasting along and there are never any challenges! It's more that the challenges evolve and grow, and people can still say unkind things.

A case in point is an incident that occurred in one of the places I worked. I had recently started, and, as had happened at other places, I had made a mistake. I had sent a quote to a potential client in pounds when I had meant dollars. This is a small difference of symbols but it had big financial implications. Thankfully, as I was new, my employer thought it was just a rookie accident that wouldn't happen again, once they'd reminded me 'to double-check my work'.

But I knew it was a dyslexic mistake. That challenges like this had haunted me my entire life and would likely continue to be a problem because I find it so hard to check my own work effectively. But instead of being honest about the support I needed, I agreed that it was an 'accident' and that I would be more diligent in the future.

Telling the truth didn't feel like an option, because saying, 'I'm dyslexic and I often make small mistakes in emails and even when I have a system I worry every day that my work isn't correct' doesn't exactly feel like the kind of thing that keeps you employed.

Surprise! The next week, I made the same mistake, losing the company more money. The next thing I knew, I was sitting in a meeting room with my boss saying to me, 'Are you lazy or are you stupid?' They didn't understand how I could have made such a basic mistake twice in two weeks. Did I not care about my work? Did I not check it? Was I not capable?

I was too terrified to admit the errors were due to my dyslexia. I had already told them I was dyslexic but they hadn't put two and two together and realised that that was the reason for me making the mistakes; they weren't spelling mistakes and, like most managers, they didn't really understand what being dyslexic means. Again, what could I say? I couldn't be confident that the same thing wouldn't happen again. Also, I was too busy hating myself to think of anything better to say, so I just apologised profusely.

In between these two incidents I had come up with an amazing idea that had made the company significantly more money than I had lost due to my mistakes. At no point in that meeting did that idea feel relevant; all the manager cared about was that I did the basics well. My idea was a nice extra, but not what they really wanted from an employee.

It was moments like these that left me saying, 'Who cares about big-picture thinking?' I just wanted my brain to be able to do the basics. I felt like my strengths weren't reliable enough for me to know what to do with them, and my challenges around 'easy' tasks were too significant for me to ever advance in my career.

I left that meeting wondering if there would ever be a job I could be good at. What successful job doesn't require writing emails? Should I give up on my dreams now and just go and find a job that my brain could manage, whatever that might be? It was soon after this event that I started Dyslexia in Adults. I realised I had no idea how to manage my dyslexia and my non-strategy of just hoping it wouldn't happen again and thinking I just needed to double-check my work was causing me so much anxiety and, frankly, not working.

I often think about this story when I am speaking to my clients and hear them say the same thing: 'Maybe I should quit this career and do something my brain can cope with', which usually means doing something they deem so simple that even *their* brain would be up to the task. This comment usually comes after years of working, when a dyslexic mistake trips them up and they think, 'What is the point in doing this job any more? My brain clearly isn't built for this life.' Often, after I have probed a little, they will share with me the ideas they had and the dyslexic strengths they displayed. But the challenges beat them down – the strengths weren't enough when they were struggling every day.

But the truth is, dyslexia will follow you everywhere you go – you can't outrun it. I promise you (because I have spoken to them), the dyslexic people working in those 'simple' jobs are sometimes struggling so much with their working memory that they wish more than anything they could be in corporate jobs, where your ideas and approach are what's valued. Everyone believes the grass is greener, but once you learn to manage your challenges it makes you feel capable and that your strengths have the space to shine. Happily, managing dyslexia is exactly what I'm going to help you with.

I hope that sharing these stories will help you realise you aren't alone. That the experiences we have had as dyslexic people make having low confidence almost inevitable, because instead of our differences being supported, we've had to struggle alone and learn to mask our realities. That the cruel comments of others further entrench our negative sense of self and make us feel like we are always an imposter who will be 'found out'. Finally, that our strengths, which can be so exciting, often feel overlooked or unimportant compared to the weight of dyslexic challenges that we were never taught to manage.

As I mentioned at the beginning of this chapter, what keeps us stuck is bottling up these experiences and the deep emotions that make us feel like a failure. Instead, by recognising the universality of these experiences, we can see it is not us but the system that is letting us down, as we weren't given any choice but to mask, work hard and hope no one noticed our dyslexia. However, now is our chance to let go of that negative sense of self and create a blank slate to allow a new, more confident approach to managing dyslexia to begin.

Common dyslexic cycles

In the sections above, I talked about the common dyslexic experiences we face that create low confidence, and how now is the opportunity to let go of them and start to shift our approach to a new, more confident way. To help this process, I'm going to share a few examples of common habits many dyslexics have that are rooted in low confidence. Hopefully you can see that although they may feel like the right choice in the moment, to keep you feeling safe, in the long term they aren't serving you.

To do this, you have to first recognise those cycles. I don't want you to feel ashamed of past experiences or like you aren't able to turn things around, but I do want you to really see that finding a way to value your dyslexia and accept your differences instead of hiding is the best path. So, let's take a look a few of the most common cycles I observe in myself and other dyslexics.

Turning down jobs or opportunities

Keeping within your comfort zone is a natural reaction when you have been constantly criticised. This sees dyslexics commonly triangulating what will keep us safe and not cause us to make too many mistakes, while also not abandoning ambition entirely.

There are different areas where this may show up:

- You completely discount entire careers or areas of work due to dyslexic challenges, even if these are areas that could have benefitted from your unique thinking.

- **Example:** I wanted to be a politician when I was younger but I was too scared to go for it because I was worried about not keeping up with the 'red box' paperwork I mentioned earlier.

- You stay within your comfort zone within your role, meaning that you don't build up the experience or knowledge to be able to move forwards with your career.
  - **Example:** A client came to work with me after turning down the opportunity to run a new initiative in her team because of the planning and organisation that would be involved in managing all the moving parts. This led to the person who took on the role hogging the spotlight with senior managers and getting promoted later that year.

- The fear of what you *can't* do guides your decisions. When you first get a promotion or opportunity, your mind goes straight to all the ways you will struggle or your challenges will be highlighted, rather than focusing on what you can do or what you will offer. You worry that stepping up to this new role might mean you get 'found out' as the imposter you feel like.
  - **Example:** A client was too scared to take on a CEO role because it would involve having to write company-wide update emails. He discounted the unique ideas he had already brought to the role.
  - **Example:** The person who messaged me on Instagram to tell me she turned down a supervisor role because of the admin involved with arranging shifts.

- You only go for promotions when you're coerced by a supportive boss or family member who reminds you why you will be capable of doing the job. Often you will have turned down opportunities in the past and will only feel you can apply for a role when you're so overqualified you could do it with your eyes closed.
  - **Example:** A client was once told by her boss that she had applied for a promotion even though she hadn't, because he could see her potential and that she was too busy being scared of the spotlight and failing to apply for the role herself.

Think of all the wasted opportunities and ideas that won't get initiated simply because millions of people are too afraid to go for a job they feel incapable of doing.

On a personal level, think about the financial implications of what holding back means. You may have heard of the 'neurodiversity tax' (for example, the cost of train tickets you have to buy twice because you didn't notice you booked one for the wrong date). But what about the neurodiversity tax we experience due to not advancing in our careers? The holidays or experiences we can't afford to go on because we are too afraid of stepping up a pay grade.

As mentioned in the introduction, when I left university, I didn't go into a graduate job. I was too scared I wouldn't keep up. Instead, I chose to take a (totally unsuitable) minimum-wage data-entry job, as it felt so 'simple' that even I could do it. So, whereas most of my friends started on decent graduate salaries, I was earning significantly less.

To break this cycle, you need to take a step back and objectively assess both your skills and the role. This can feel hard when you've spent years focusing on what you can't do. So, make it visual: write a list of tasks required by the role, then colour-code them. Use green for things you will be good at, orange for tasks you may need more support with, and red for where you see challenges. Really push yourself to be objective when choosing orange and red. The visual overview might help you see the truth of how minimal the areas you struggle with actually are, and how valuable your strengths could be for the role. You can then also use the information to ask for more support or training.

Putting yourself down/never taking a compliment

I bet I'm right when I say that I don't think you take compliments well. Perhaps you brush them off or minimise them with phrases like, 'Even a wrong clock is right twice a day.' Maybe you're unable to look past the struggles and see your value, essentially viewing your challenges as 'you' and any successes as 'a fluke'.

This deep-rooted feeling of not being capable and being unable to accept that you're good at something is common in people with dyslexia. You're so used to struggling, that when something comes easily, it gets discounted. The negativity seeps in over time; as your confidence is eroded, you don't realise how much it impacts you and how long you have been feeling bad about yourself.

Perception is reality. If you spend the whole time saying you are disorganised or useless, don't be surprised when someone thinks that about you.

You may think being able to take a compliment is a minor matter, but minimising your success by immediately undermining the compliment prevents others from seeing how capable you truly are. People believe what you tell them, so you need to be careful not to create an unhelpful narrative.

To break this cycle, you need to stop feeling that dyslexia makes you an imposter who is going to be 'found out'. For many of us, those little self-deprecating jokes are a window into what we truly feel about ourselves. It can be easy to think that if you put it out there first then you are controlling the narrative or managing expectations so no one is surprised when there is a slip-up. But it's time to start challenging those thoughts, not letting imposter syndrome run rampant in your head. This requires you to look back at past achievements, and to acknowledge that you have come this far and you are more capable than you believe.

Catastrophising mistakes

When you make a spelling mistake as a dyslexic, you aren't just berating yourself for that one slip-up: your mind goes to the thousands of times it has happened before. This reminds you of:

- People laughing at you for the silly ways you spell things.
- The countless times your homework came back covered in red pen.
- The hundreds of times even spellcheck couldn't understand you.

The weight of those thousands of other mistakes, and the reaction they got, all feeds into the narrative that you aren't capable. But not seeing the situation as a stand-alone moment means you aren't able to analyse it objectively and build better approaches. To illustrate this point, here's an example of the same scenario, viewed two different ways:

Situation: you make a spelling mistake in an important email.

1) Catastrophised version:

'How could I be so useless?'

'They are going to think I can't even write a simple email.'

'I don't know why I am even in this job if I can't write an email to senior managers.'

2) Viewing the situation as an isolated moment:

'OK, that mistake wasn't great, but at least the rest of the email contains good ideas and they will understand what I said.'

'That mistake slipped through because I was doing too many tasks at once. I need to build a system to only do important checking work when I am not flustered.'

In this situation, it's important to understand that hating yourself doesn't help you build better systems – it just keeps you in a cycle of struggle.

To break this cycle, you need to learn how to stop catastrophising mistakes and look at them in a more realistic way. Our mistakes are often not that significant and don't need to be something that sends us into a negative spiral or defines us. From now on, dyslexic mistakes need to be molehills, not mountains. By viewing your challenges in this way, you will be able to see where you are capable and where you need to build simple strategies for improvement, rather than keeping the cycle going and feeling useless and hoping hard work will help you catch the mistake next time.

4
How to grow in confidence

> **Chapter summary**
>
> **Why this chapter is important**
>
> The previous chapter was all about how and why your confidence may have been knocked, but now it's time to work on rebuilding it. This all starts with owning and accepting your difference and understanding why it's so important. We'll then take a look at low-confidence habits – what they are and how to unlearn them – as well as strategies to build your confidence, both now and in the future.
>
> **What you will learn**
> - Why shame, denial and masking are so damaging.
> - How to view your dyslexia as a difference that's neutral – neither good nor bad.
> - How owning your dyslexia can be beneficial.
> - How to break the cycle of low confidence.
> - How to build a pathway to gaining confidence.

I know dwelling on the negative experiences of dyslexia can feel uncomfortable and chapter 3 might have felt like a call-out for many of you, but this book is about practical solutions, so let's talk about how to build confidence.

First, we're going to look at how to accept being dyslexic, and different – as it's by owning and accepting your difference that we can move to a place where we can implement strategies that will help us.

Second, I will explain how to break the cycle of low confidence and the bad habits you have likely adopted. Even if you have already done some work on your confidence, you may still have some lingering 'low-confidence habits': thinking you're useless, that everything is going to go wrong, that you've made a mistake, etc. These are often deeply entrenched and require a lot of unpicking.

Third, I'll give you some strategies to help you gain in confidence.

It's all about acceptance

When I talk about 'growing in confidence', I mean the confidence that comes not just from implementing good strategies, but from accepting that you are dyslexic and not trying to hide it.

Stopping masking and starting to work with your difference can feel really scary due to the shame of past experiences. I know this, but what I hope I showed in chapter 3 is that, although it is scary, so is continuing with the same approach, since that isn't working either.

To put it bluntly, masking has repercussions:

- **Challenges are made even harder**
  Instead of putting in place strategies that work and enable us to do things differently, we adopt ones that hide our dyslexia, meaning that tasks take longer and you feel your output doesn't reflect your effort.

- **Strengths are undervalued by you**
  Because you're so busy working on your challenges, often only by working harder, you aren't able to put time and effort into your strengths. This means they are not nurtured and the opportunities they could bring aren't realised.

- **Your confidence is undermined**
  Often, a bar is set and tasks are deemed 'easy' or 'difficult' based on a neurotypical person's perception. This means that when you as a dyslexic person are unable to reach that bar you feel useless. This inevitably makes you question your competence and berate yourself, focusing solely on your challenges and losing confidence in your other abilities.

This cycle of struggling with challenges, undervaluing strengths and losing confidence in yourself can last a lifetime. It can also be very damaging and have a broad impact on your life and work. Often, all it takes is a small shift in your equilibrium for the whole house of cards to come crashing down. This might be triggered by events such as becoming a parent and having less time to deal with challenges, or a boss or person in a position of power being particularly picky. These small shifts in your situation can turn dyslexia from a challenge into a huge issue that upends your life. So, how do we break this cycle? The goal is to change our thinking and understand and accept that dyslexia makes us different. This is neither good nor bad; it's just different.

Setting a new goal of seeing dyslexia as a neutral difference can, for many, be an easier stepping stone than reaching the high bar of superpower. My concern is that if we are given a binary choice between toxic positivity and negative feelings, it can be easier to stay in the negative. So by offering a third way – seeing dyslexia as a difference that brings both challenges and strengths, in the same way *everyone* has weaknesses and strengths – we can start to move away from the negative view.

It is through this acceptance of dyslexia being a neutral difference that we stop putting our effort into learning how to be 'normal' and masking our challenges, and instead focus on building strategies to unlock dyslexia and create successful habits and structures in our lives. This acceptance means we end the constant reaching for a version of ourselves that isn't dyslexic – an impossible goal that erodes confidence because you can't be the version of yourself that you want to be.

What neutral looks like

Dyslexia brings with it both challenges and huge value. It is the root of many of your struggles and the path for most of your opportunities.

1. **Owning the challenges**

   It is OK to acknowledge and accept that dyslexia can cause significant challenges that impact your life, but the key here is to realise that everyone has challenges and that these just happen to be yours. Despite what others have said about you in the past, often the mistakes you make are very minor in the grand scheme of things. For more on this, see 'Catastrophising mistakes' on p. 57.

   To deal with these challenges, you need to operate in a way that is different to others. That different style can frustrate them – but that's their problem, not yours. To jump off the struggle treadmill and truly start feeling capable, you need to advocate for what you need in order to succeed. This is covered in much more detail in section 2, which is packed with strategies and advice.

2. **Owning the value**

   Understand that your challenges do not detract from your strengths. Your unique ideas and abilities have real value and can bring great opportunity into your life. Often we can get bogged down in our challenges and skim over our successes, but try to see them as separate and give your successes the celebration they deserve. For example, if you get your timings wrong and turn up late to a panel talk but wow the audience with your amazing ideas, you don't need to repeatedly say, 'Sorry I was late' – enjoy the success and let the slip-up melt away. This is something we go into in more detail in section 3.

Real-world story

Sometimes, it can be a lot easier outside of work to see how to manage dyslexia in a different way, as there is less pressure and the impact of us trying something new is less obvious. Let me give you an example of how in my personal life I have owned the value of my strengths and accepted the reality of my challenges.

I am confident my dyslexia makes me a great friend: I'm incredibly supportive and good at providing advice and ideas when it comes to friends' problems. However, that doesn't mean I don't make mistakes – I'm only human!

I've spent hours with close friends talking through problems in their lives. They have often said that I am able to see the issue from multiple sides and can offer suggestions they wouldn't have thought of. Not only do I feel proud that my dyslexic strengths have been valuable to my friends, but I have also heard many juicy stories! You've got to take the wins where you can!

However, for all that I love and care about my friends and family, I will at some point have forgotten their birthday. I might remember a few days later, but it's definitely something I struggle with due to my dyslexia. I can forgive myself for this. Given the choice between always being able to recall every birthday on time or being able to provide valued advice, I know which one I'd choose every time.

Real-world story

Recently, a client came to me seeking help so that she could spend less time checking and double-checking her reports. Her job was to be involved in diagnosing people with neurodiversity, using an ever-evolving landscape of new tools and ideas. This meant each report would take longer to do as she cross-checked the various papers. One of her main fears was that she was forgetting something important, but she was also embarrassed at the time it took her to do this work and felt like she wasn't pulling her weight to help the department reduce the ever-growing backlog.

Our strategy was quite simple: rather than focusing on her frustrations, we took some time to work through and put all the important information into a single digestible document so she could review all the reports against one central source of information. This strategy would serve to support working memory management and make good use of her strengths in terms of creating the big picture.

When we discussed when she was going to get this done, she said she wanted to do it in her own time. In her mind, because she was 'already a burden to the team', she couldn't take more time during work hours to do it. I asked her if she thought other people in her team also struggled with this issue of having to cross-refer against several documents. She said it always came up in team meetings and was a common problem.

I reminded her that one of her key goals was to improve her confidence and instead of seeing the task as a 'burden' she had to take on, she should view it as a project that would help the entire team. She spoke to her team lead and offered to share the document around after she'd finished it, during work

> hours. The team were so grateful for the document and for her explanation of how to create a version of their own if they wanted to, and for the fact that she would update it consistently in the future.
>
> In this example, owning her dyslexia meant that instead of being ashamed of the challenge, my client was excited by the opportunity to build a better system that could support the whole team.

The goal

Take a step back and see yourself as a fully rounded person instead of zooming in on every tiny mistake and wasting time and energy wishing your brain worked differently. Yes, the challenges are real, but so are the strengths that you offer. Hating yourself won't help you manage the challenges or unlock the strengths.

Why owning your dyslexia works

I'm not saying owning your dyslexia doesn't mean you'll never face another negative comment or experience, but it's the only way to reach your potential, unlock your strengths, and make your challenges more manageable.

I like to visualise dyslexia as a backpack. You're already carrying it around, and every challenge – such as working memory issues, executive function difficulties or slow processing speed – adds another brick. Then come the confidence bricks: overworking to prove yourself, putting yourself down, hiding your strengths. Every time you pile one of those on top, you increase the load, when you're already overloaded.

By choosing to own your dyslexia and let go of the shame you have about your negative habits, you shed some of that weight. This frees up time and energy to focus on what you're good at, and helps you start to manage your challenges more effectively. This makes everything feel a bit easier – and your experience of being dyslexic becomes more neutral.

How owning your dyslexia can be beneficial

1. It allows you to understand and use legal protections

In the UK The Equality Act 2010 is an incredible piece of legislation that offers strong protections to neurodiverse people. I believe that when we accept dyslexia as a neutral fact – not something to be ashamed of – we become better at asking for accommodations and standing up for ourselves when our rights are ignored.

Sadly, most dyslexic people internalise discrimination. We see ourselves as a 'burden' or 'problem' to fix, especially when we lack strategies or support. Toxic workplaces then feel like our fault, and we worry we're asking for 'too much'.

Many of my clients only realise – once they've built confidence – how minor their challenges actually are, and how small the accommodations they needed were. Yet across our lifetimes and regularly at work we had been made to feel that our challenges were too big to support or that our requests for help were too unrealistic.

> **Real-world story**
>
> Recently, I spoke at a dyslexia conference. The speaker after me – a lawyer – shared how powerful the Equality Act is, and how it can help people feel confident asking for support and rejecting discrimination.
>
> I sat for over an hour, listening to hundreds of dyslexics share similar stories: workplace challenges, ignored needs and repeated violations of the law by companies. It was infuriating.
>
> And I realised my story was just like everyone else's. I'd apologised to people who spoke to me rudely. I'd accepted

> unlawful treatment. My probation had been extended multiple times, and no one had cared that I was dyslexic – they just expected me to be the same as everyone else. I was even asked to leave one of the world's largest companies without being offered any reasonable adjustments, even though I'd told them my challenges were due to dyslexia.
>
> It makes me so angry – both for myself and for millions of others – how our perspective has hindered our ability to get what we need and deserve.

What is The Equality Act 2010? This act was introduced in the UK to protect disabled people and promote access through reasonable adjustments. Neurodiversity wasn't specifically named back in 2010, but it has since been included.

'Reasonable adjustments' mean changes that an employer, education provider or service provider can make to support access. The Act doesn't list specific adjustments – which can be frustrating – but that vagueness is intentional. It allows for individual circumstances to be considered, rather than setting prescriptive rules.

Most neurodiverse people don't realise how much is considered reasonable. I've been shocked by how broad the protections are – especially for large organisations, who might struggle to argue that something isn't reasonable.

Here are some examples of adjustments that you might think are 'too much' but are actually perfectly reasonable:

- Using an automatic car instead of a manual.
- Flexible work hours or arriving late.
- Receiving interview questions in advance.
- Expecting timely installation of assistive technology.

How to grow in confidence

> **Kumulchew v Starbucks**
>
> One of my favourite cases is Kumulchew v Starbucks. A dyslexic employee was fired for 'falsifying' documents – but the mistakes were due to difficulties with numbers. The court found that Starbucks failed to provide reasonable accommodations to manage this challenge.

The sad truth is, many people have been treated atrociously and said nothing – partly because they didn't know the law was on their side, but also because they saw dyslexia as a 'problem' they had to fix. When you believe that, it's easier to accept poor treatment – or worse, *expect* it.

So, instead of recognising injustice and fighting back, what I see over and over again is that we just move jobs again, lose confidence, and keep trying to prove to ourselves and others that we are capable. But that doubt should never have existed in the first place.

> **How to ask for reasonable adjustments**
>
> The Equality Act 2010 applies in the UK, but other countries have different laws and legislations to give provisions for those who need them. Do your research and find out what your rights are.
>
> Wherever you live, if you believe your rights are being breached – especially in the workplace – the first step is to raise the issue. In some cases, the organisation may genuinely be unaware of their legal obligations, though employers are expected to know the law and cannot use ignorance as a defence.
>
> You should clearly state that you're dyslexic (and mention any other neurodivergence, if relevant), and request reasonable adjustments that would help you access your role and environment more effectively. These adjustments should be

tailored to your needs and ideally supported by examples or evidence (such as a diagnostic report or occupational health assessment), though this is not always required.

Under The Equality Act 2010:

- Employers and service providers have a legal duty to consider reasonable adjustments once they are aware (or should be reasonably aware) of a disability.
- They must either implement the adjustments or provide clear, evidence-based reasons why a specific adjustment is not considered reasonable in their context.
- Failure to do so many constitute unlawful discrimination.

Let me say this plainly: we are collectively making a mistake. Years of negative experiences have made us feel like we're a burden. That deep drive to prove we're 'normal' is exactly what is holding us back.

It's time to feel deserving of support. To be shocked when discrimination happens. And to take people to court when they break the law.

2. You can focus on what works for you

Dyslexic people can do any job. I don't say this just because I want it to be true – I say it because I've spoken to dyslexic people in every kind of role you can think of, including the ones most people wrongly assume are off-limits.

Here are just a few examples of dyslexic professionals I've worked with who have roles that don't fit the stereotypical mould:

- Consultants at major firms
- Lawyers handling complex cases
- GPs
- Senior genetic consultants
- Criminal forensic specialists

- Senior civil servants
- Executive assistants to senior executives
- Senior scientists leading large research projects
- CEOs

These individuals were adding real value and making a success of their careers, in their own dyslexic way.

There's no 'impossible' or 'shouldn't' about it – it's about understanding yourself and where you would best shine rather than building a life around 'can't' and comparing yourself to others.

Real-world story

One of my clients was a department head within a hospital. He had worked hard and was respected by his colleagues and the senior leadership team alike. His team valued his ideas and his ability to solve complex cases – he'd even developed innovative systems to manage patient backlogs, which was critical for improving patient care.

But he couldn't see any of that.

Instead, he focused on how frustrated he got with the daily flow of emails and case notes, feeling embarrassed by his 'failure' to manage the routine admin. His role had evolved to focus more on department strategy and structural improvements, yet he still felt useless because in his mind 'he couldn't manage the basics'.

I get so frustrated by the idea that there is a 'perfect' job for dyslexic people. I don't believe that.

What we need to talk about instead are the working styles and cultures that fail dyslexic people. When we accept our dyslexia and understand our needs, we realise that not every workplace will suit us – and that's OK. It's not a flaw to be different. It's not a failure to walk away from environments that don't support you.

I constantly tell clients who are job-hunting: the best thing you can do for your career is accept that you shouldn't work for most companies. You are valuable. Your strengths matter. The goal is to find a place where those strengths can flourish.

> **Out of the frying pan and into the fire**
>
> A common pattern I see is this: a dyslexic person struggles with a particular job in a toxic workplace that amplifies their challenges. They leave quickly – understandably – but then rush into the next job out of desperation.
>
> In that rush, they ignore red flags in interviews. They just hope things will be better this time. But without taking the time to reflect on what they actually need, they end up in another environment that fails them – sometimes worse than the last.
>
> The cycle continues, not because they're not capable, but because they haven't been given the space to understand what kind of workplace allows them to feel successful.

3. You learn to spot, and respond to, red flags

There is nothing worse than a toxic workplace. It drains you. By the time you quit, you're a shell of yourself. Before that, you're dragging yourself home feeling useless, worrying about the next day. Your whole week becomes a countdown for the weekend, and even then, Sunday morning hits and you're already dreading Monday. That leaves just one day a week when you can breathe easy. I wouldn't wish it on my worst enemy – I've been there.

Deep down, I knew my brain didn't fit the mould at the places I worked at. I never believed I was incapable, but many managers made me feel this way when I couldn't do tasks their way – and anything different meant I was 'less than'. It regularly made my life miserable.

Here is the flip side: dyslexic people can be successful in any role and lead in any field – if they're allowed to work differently. That requires a supportive manager. That one simple fact can change everything.

So notice and respond to the red flags. Watch for those moments in interviews when the boss seems inflexible or the company's expectations are clearly unreasonable. Don't ignore these warning signs – run for the hills!

Every job that turned into a nightmare for me? I knew from the start. My dyslexic intuition clocked it. Yet I ignored it, believing pig-headedly I would be fine and I could push through. If only I'd admitted to myself that it's OK to find certain tasks difficult – and it's better to have support from the beginning. Instead, for most of my working life, admitting that felt like giving in to my deepest fear.

Now, I help clients rigorously assess companies – and particularly managers – to help them understand how they can do their best in a particular role. Because that's what companies want: your best. They just don't always realise that for that to happen, you need to do things differently.

When I was struggling, I used to believe I could push through any bad situation and it was my responsibility to learn how to work in any circumstance. Now, I focus on what I am good at and am clear on how bad systems impact me. If I were to apply for a job again, I wouldn't work for just anyone or in any company. I know that I'd need to choose the right role for me carefully. That would mean paying attention to the red flags and avoiding bosses who'd be unsympathetic and cause more stress than I could handle.

Bad systems let dyslexic people fall through the gaps. I've coached many dyslexic clients who began by telling me that they were the problem – that they needed to learn how to process faster or improve their skills. But when we dug into specific examples of what had happened that made them feel like that, often what emerged was a system or company culture that was so unrealistic or rigid that it was the bad system failing the dyslexic person, not the dyslexic person failing the system.

Other members of staff may have raised similar frustrations and concerns, but the intensity of the impact on dyslexic individuals – and our deep desire to be capable – led my clients to internalise the problem. They believed they *were* the problem, when in fact they were falling through the cracks of a bad system.

You're just trying to do your best

When we start to view dyslexia as a neutral difference, it can help us realise that utilising strategies and approaching life through the lens of being different isn't about listing deficits as an excuse. Instead it is about saying, 'Here is what I need support with or what I need to approach differently, so I can do my best and be successful for you.' It's about realising that getting support is about setting you up for success, because masking doesn't minimise challenges – it makes them worse.

It is about channelling the hard-working ethos that dyslexia has instilled in us into something more positive. You are putting effort into showing up and being the best version of yourself rather than sitting in shame and hoping it will be better next week, even though you know that is unlikely.

4. You won't waste time wishing you weren't dyslexic

Accepting that this is the only brain you'll ever have – even if you never tell anyone you are dyslexic – can be a turning point. It was for me, and it's helped many of my clients as well. It's easy to glance around an office and wish you were like your colleagues, but that kind of thinking doesn't make the situation any easier.

There will, of course, be people who may be quicker at certain tasks than you or able to do other things that you find difficult, but there is always another side to the coin. If someone's highly detail-oriented, they'll likely find it harder to see the big picture and all the benefits that come with that (as discussed in chapter 15).

I often tell people: the very thing you overlook in yourself is often what others wish they had.

When you admire that detail-oriented person, I promise you – they're admiring your ability to transcend the minutiae and spot patterns, connections and opportunities.

One of my closest friends is brilliant with detail. I am constantly impressed by how she never misses things, forgets appointments or turns up late. These are all areas I have to manage with active strategies – and even then, I slip up occasionally. I used to think she was 'better than me', more competent at managing life. But she regularly reminds me how much she values my ability to see the big picture, and how she wishes she could do what I do.

It's not that either one of these strengths is 'better'. Each strength has its own value. Ironically, we spent years wishing we had each other's abilities, without realising how much we already brought to the table.

How to break the cycle of low confidence

I never believed I would be a confident person – so if I can do it, so can you. These days, I proudly ask for accommodations and very rarely find myself loathing my brain. I say 'rarely' because there is the odd time when I catch myself falling into old habits. But I catch myself quicker now, and I no longer shrink away from challenges because of dyslexia.

The strategies that changed my entire life have helped my clients, too. They've shown that hating dyslexia or wishing your brain worked differently don't help. Some strategies are quick wins; others take time to build. But all are tried and tested, and they work. They help you shed the shame and stand tall in your difference – embracing both the challenges and the strengths.

It all starts with shifting how you think about dyslexia, because the foundation of confidence is seeing your difference as something neutral, and definitely not something to be ashamed of. That shift affects how you talk about it, how you hold yourself, how you manage it, and how you communicate and speak up. And those are the markers of a confident dyslexic person.

Who decides which tasks are easy?

The time you spend sitting and loathing yourself is eating up valuable headspace. It's time to stop believing that one spelling mistake in an important email makes you useless at everything else.

There's a list of tasks that dyslexic people often struggle with – yet society has labelled them 'easy'. That label doesn't help. It feeds the internal narrative that your brain is broken because it can't even handle something 'simple'.

> **But here's the key point: if it's difficult *for you*, then it's difficult. Reclassify it as such.**

Take getting up to speed on a new project, for example. Understanding all the new elements of a task and feeling clear on what the expectations are can be difficult. It catches you out, crunches your timings and leaves you frustrated. If you treat this as an 'easy' task, you'll keep guessing and miscalculating. But if you recognise it as a genuine challenge, you'll start breaking tasks down more effectively and feel more comfortable asking for support. Taking these challenges seriously, even just privately, can make a huge difference to your success.

So seriously – who decided these tasks were easy? They're not – at least not for you and me. Next time you find yourself getting frustrated because you can't do a 'simple' task, I want you to challenge that negative thought. Remind yourself that it's not easy for over 700 million dyslexic people.

And remember: the things *we* find easy are often the very things others label as 'difficult'. It's not just our challenges that need recognition – our strengths do, too.

Low-value v high-value tasks

This is one of my favourite confidence-boosting concepts for dyslexic people: we need to reclassify tasks. As I mentioned above, we find some 'easy' tasks hard, and vice versa. Instead of thinking in terms of 'easy' and 'hard' and obsessing over micro-mistakes, change your perspective. Think in terms of low-value tasks v high-value tasks.

Low-value tasks – these are everyday admin tasks. If they go wrong, it's frustrating – but not the end of the world. Examples include:

- Forgetting to attach a document to an email.
- Sending an invitation with the wrong date.
- Forgetting cheese at the supermarket even though your partner reminded you five times.

High-value tasks – these are tasks that are transformative and long-lasting. They change people's lives, revolutionise companies and make teams more efficient. Examples include:

- Spotting a recurring pain point and creating a new product.
- Anticipating problems and making proactive changes.

- Bringing initiatives from another industry or field into your role or situation to create efficiencies.
- Recognising the need for a community hub or awareness campaign that will benefit vulnerable members of the community.

You have to flip the script. Most people see low-value tasks as easy and high-value tasks as hard. But for most dyslexic people, it's the opposite. High-value thinking comes naturally. Low-value admin can be a minefield.

When you think about it from that perspective and truly add up what your high-value thinking has contributed – to your life, your work, your relationships – you'll start to see the opportunity in dyslexia. Confidence grows when you realise there's nothing wrong with your difference. It's just that what you find easy and difficult is different from others – and that difference has huge value.

Real-world story

I had a coaching client come to me feeling insecure, confused and deeply frustrated with how his brain worked. His confidence had repeatedly been knocked and he was feeling drained by constant negative feedback.

When we started discussing why he had such low confidence in himself, he said that his writing had been consistently criticised. Across the board, small errors had been pointed out in his emails, presentations and reports, which had made people think he wasn't checking his work properly.

We worked on strategies for checking his own work, and then to improve his confidence I introduced him to the concept of low-value v high-value tasks. I explained that spelling everything perfectly is a low-value task. Yes, it's frustrating when a mistake slips through, but people still understand what you mean. It's rarely catastrophic.

Then I asked him to name a high-value contribution he'd made to his role. His low confidence meant his first reply was, 'I'm not sure I'm good at anything.' But with a little probing, he revealed something extraordinary: he had recently suggested a new process that was saving the company so much time that he had been given a large pay rise.

He hadn't had to sit in a day-long strategy workshop on time management and he wasn't the team manager whose job it was to think about workplace efficiency, he'd simply spotted inefficiencies and proposed a solution. His ability to see the big picture led to a change that helped an entire team operate more effectively while also reducing their workload.

However, he was so focused on the constant low-value challenges that he'd decided should be easy that his confidence had been undermined and he couldn't see the huge benefit he had brought with his high-value ideas.

How to silence the voice in your head

Years of negative experiences can build a narrative in our minds that we're 'useless' in certain areas. For dyslexic people, this internal voice often runs unchecked. But stopping those thoughts running free in your mind is essential to creating change.

Here is the mental picture I like to paint for my clients:

Your mind is a tennis court. You are standing on one side, and the ball machine is on the other. It's firing negative thoughts at you. Right now, you're doing nothing. The balls are piling up, and you're tripping over them.

Next time the machine starts, pick up your racket and start hitting those balls back over to the other side of the net. Because otherwise, letting negative thoughts build up will keep you stuck in a cycle of low confidence.

Here are a few mental swings I like to use:

- 'Hating myself doesn't help.'
- 'This mistake isn't the end of the world – it doesn't change how they understand my work.'
- 'This is just a bad system I need to improve; it doesn't make me incapable.'

The goal isn't to eliminate all the negative comments, but to challenge them in the moment. Put them into context. Don't let them spiral into catastrophes.

Don't try to fix every element of dyslexia

Dyslexia comes with daily moments that can feel hugely embarrassing, but our job is to figure out what is a challenge that needs strategies and what isn't a big deal and is in fact something that we just need to move on from. Spending every second fussing and worrying about all the micro-moments kills your confidence, and trying to avoid minor issues eats up hours of your life.

There are some times in life when we need the perfectly written document – for example, you wouldn't want your name spelled wrong on a marriage licence – but there are other moments when a small slip-up isn't the end of the world, such as saying 'your' when you meant 'you're' in a WhatsApp message.

Not every frustration needs a solution. Sometimes, radical acceptance is the most effective way to manage your neurodiversity.

For clients who are struggling with multiple frustrations, I ask them to make a list of challenges they're willing to accept – without shame or self-punishment. Here are a few of mine:

- Forgetting to attach important documents to emails (resending quickly isn't that embarrassing).
- Spelling mistakes in texts to friends (if they understand me, what does it matter?).
- Needing accountability or body doubling for difficult tasks (sometimes ADHD makes achieving difficult tasks frustrating and needing someone to chat to you while you do it isn't a failure – it's a strategy).

Stop trying to prove yourself

Dyslexia often creates a gap between what you're capable of and what your output shows. This can lead to years of overwork, trying to prove you're capable – while fearing you're not.

This need to prove yourself shows up in many ways:

1. **Feeling like a burden**

    Many of my clients know what support works for them. They've even tried my strategies before. But they don't use them consistently because they fear that asking for help makes them a burden. In reality, avoiding making adjustments often leads to bigger, costlier mistakes. Feeling like a burden doesn't help you succeed – it keeps you stuck in a cycle of struggling and can result in underperforming.

    This type of thinking is not helpful for growing confidence. Instead, we need to realise that small changes can make a big difference. Most people around you want you to do your best and succeed. A few tweaks in how you work won't make you a burden but they will make you significantly more successful.

2. **Not using systems**

    As I mentioned above, some dyslexic people work late into the night or at weekends to hide their differences and need for support. This is unsustainable and unnecessary. As we discussed on p. 64, it's time to see systems as you wanting to do your best, not as a sign of being incapable.

3. **Believing 'tomorrow will be better'**
I often tell people who are struggling with dyslexia: the mystical land of 'tomorrow' doesn't exist. Hoping that tomorrow you'll work harder and magically make fewer mistakes simply won't happen.

Grit and grind have got you far, but using tried-and-tested strategies will get you further. But strategies need confidence. I can give you every strategy under the sun but if you don't have confidence to advocate for yourself and your needs then they won't work.

Which is why confidence and strategies go hand in hand. You need the confidence to start using the strategies and once they start working, your confidence will grow. So often, the hardest part of getting started is letting go of the idea that hiding your differences and working harder will fix everything. It won't. But putting strategies in place will.

> ## Real-world story
>
> Recently, I've worked with many clients in the public sector, where workloads are unmanageable and expectations stretch far beyond what's realistic. One woman came to me convinced that her dyslexia was the problem and she believed that she needed to learn to manage her dyslexia better to fit the expectations of her role in the police.
>
> But after a few sessions – in which we broke down exactly what she wanted to achieve and what she hoped would be possible –

> she began to see things differently. The problem wasn't her dyslexia: it was the role itself.
>
> She would often say in our sessions, 'I know dyslexia makes it harder, but the truth is this job is unreasonable – and I never realised that before.' She was so busy focusing on feeling like a burden, she couldn't actually look at the role and figure out what was reasonable and what wasn't.
>
> Once we got rid of all the negative emotions that stopped her from thinking clearly, we were able to get specific about areas that could make her life easier and help her feel like she was in control of how she was managing her dyslexia.

Pathway to creating confidence

There are lots of ways to improve and grow your confidence but when dyslexia is at the root of the issue, we must address the underlying cause, not just the symptoms. Here are two foundational steps to restoring dyslexic confidence and navigating the realities of dyslexic life without further eroding your self-belief.

1. **Confidence needs to be worked on**

    It sounds obvious, but confidence doesn't just occur because you sent an email without a spelling mistake or went a week without a dyslexic challenge. It doesn't even reliably show up when your boss accepts an idea you had and is running with it, or when someone you love reminds you of your worth.

    Confidence lives deeper than that. It's built at your core – we have to believe that our dyslexia isn't something to be ashamed of. We have to work hard to change the mindset that may have been drilled into us through the thousands of negative experiences or comments we have received.

I always think in stories, so here's the image I use with clients. Your confidence is a small island in the middle of the ocean. The waves crashing against its shores are people's comments and your lived experiences. Over time, they erode the land. Your job is to rebuild the shoreline and put up defences against future erosion.

This island constantly requires protecting and working on. It doesn't stay the same and will continue to ebb and flow based on how harsh the waters are around us. It is our job to protect our island – to guard against surrounding waters becoming too damaging, and to stop the sand from being so easily washed away.

That might be about changing your perceptions about situations or changing your environment. Either way, seeing your island as something that needs tending and caring for is important.

To continue this metaphor, I think it's important to work at the edges of your island, not just the centre, where we feel most comfortable. If you don't protect the perimeter, the sturdy centre will soon be at risk. This means pushing yourself in areas that may feel uncomfortable. If there is something causing shame in your life, you need to develop a strategy to manage it, rather than ignoring or avoiding it.

2. **Learn how to be different**
Why would you put yourself out there and push yourself if you don't have good systems? If you don't feel in control of your brain, it's hard to feel confident being different.

The best way to handle being different is to understand your brain and build systems that support it. Learning about and understanding dyslexia is the most important step towards feeling capable and in control. Only then can you stop keeping yourself small and start to stretch yourself.

Examples of low-confidence habits – and mindset shifts to break them

Confidence starts with how you feel about yourself and how you feel about your dyslexia. But it deepens through action – how you hold yourself, how you speak. I often say confidence is like a good lemon drizzle cake: you need the lemon all the way down to the bottom. So every small action you take is your opportunity to poke little holes and let the confidence soak through.

I have noticed that many dyslexics develop low-confidence habits that start as coping mechanisms but become ingrained behaviours. Here's how to spot them, shift them and adopt the mindset that makes change possible:

1. Staying quiet in meetings

The low-confidence habit: Again and again I see working memory challenges stopping dyslexic people from speaking up and engaging in meetings. The difficulty in keeping up or ordering complex thoughts means it feels easier to stay quiet rather than saying something and risking embarrassing yourself.

The shift I recommend: We discuss working memory in detail in chapter 9, but the simple message is: don't try to hold everything in your head. Focus on retaining only key chunks of information. This makes it easier to process and break down thoughts.

The mindset shift that makes it possible: Your ideas are your most valuable asset and staying quiet due to fears of how you communicate is one of the most fundamental mistakes we can make as dyslexic people.

2. Keeping your ideas to yourself

The low-confidence habit: Many dyslexic people tell me they had a great idea but they didn't present it due to fear that 'someone would have thought of that' or there 'must be a reason it's done that way'. This stems from a lack of trust in our brains, meaning we don't believe in our strengths and it can feel scary or uncomfortable to share an idea.

The shift I recommend: Start to pay attention to your dyslexic strengths and the feedback you get about your ideas and way of thinking. Instead of dismissing them, it's important to acknowledge how often you may have been right – this builds trust in your own brain and will give you confidence next time an idea strikes.

The mindset shift that makes it possible: One idea or concept can have huge impact and be valuable in ways you can't even imagine. Our ideas often speak louder than our challenges, so don't rob yourself of that opportunity.

3. Struggling in silence

The low-confidence habit: Often, dyslexic people feel like asking for support makes you a burden, and that it's easier to struggle silently because you've 'managed OK so far'.

The shift I recommend: Use the 80:20 rule (*see* p. 121). You're already doing most of the work. Seeking support is not as much work as you think – and doing so prevents bigger mistakes.

The mindset shift that makes it possible: When you ask for support, you're only trying to do the best you can. Your task (in the workplace, at least) is to try to achieve a goal for someone else – so you deserve the tools to do it well. Struggling in silence doesn't serve anyone.

4. Avoiding opportunities

The low-confidence habit: Sadly, I commonly speak to people who have not applied for promotions, gone for dream careers or pushed themselves because they feel that a stretch role would highlight their dyslexia. It is easier to play safe and stay small.

The shift I recommend: When assessing an opportunity, instead of thinking about your dyslexia and all the reasons you would struggle, make sure you also make a list of reasons your dyslexia might make you capable or valuable in that role.

The mindset shift that makes it possible: Dyslexia requires strategies. It doesn't matter what job you do or what industry you work in: there will always be dyslexic challenges. There is no 'perfect' job or situation for dyslexics, only the right environment. If you have that, anything is possible.

5
Maintaining confidence in the long term

Chapter summary

Why this chapter is important

It's all very well rebuilding confidence, but how do you maintain it in the face of continuing challenges? This chapter takes a look at some of the practical things we can do to preserve our self-belief and stop others from bringing us crashing back down.

What you will learn

- How to be more selective about jobs and roles that will work for you, not against you.
- How to change your mindset about mistakes, and turn them into opportunities for change.
- How to stop belittling yourself.
- How to stop others being negative about you.
- How to implement change at work.

Simple changes to protect confidence

We know the world isn't built for dyslexic brains. Tasks labelled 'easy' often take us longer or are difficult to achieve without support. This means that despite rebuilding confidence, new situations can still knock us off course. This chapter is all about how to protect yourself from those moments and maintain confidence over time.

Only put yourself where you are valued

Moving forwards, it's essential to avoid roles that don't value your strengths. Just because you can't succeed in one environment doesn't mean you won't find another place that sees your inherent value and is excited by what you have to offer.

Flip the narrative. Instead of thinking 100 per cent of jobs should work for you, reframe it: maybe only 20 per cent of jobs truly suit your thinking style. That's not a limitation – it's a strength. You're looking for the right fit, not trying to squeeze into the wrong one. It's a privilege for someone to work with you. You're here to shine, not wither. Not again!

This means spotting red flags (*see* p. 71) and recognising that you'll still be dyslexic whether or not you disclose it. The challenges and opportunities remain the same. So ask yourself:

- Is this workplace the right environment for me?
- Is it open to new approaches and willing to be open-minded?
- Will they value my ideas and offer additional support? For example, would they see email-checking assistance as a no-brainer?

These workplaces exist. And once you're in one, your strengths will be valued, your challenges will be seen as reasonable and supported, and you'll be free to do your job to the best of your ability. I know it sounds simple, but it starts with choosing an environment that allows you to feel successful, rather than one that forces you to fight against yourself and your challenges every day.

See mistakes not as a failure but as a need for a system change

Next time you make a mistake that is connected to dyslexia, don't drown in shame. Don't tell yourself you're not capable or didn't try hard enough. Instead, see it as a sign that the system or strategy isn't working – and make changes for next time.

As discussed earlier, stop believing in the mystical land of 'tomorrow' where things magically improve. What works is changing the system.

Review past situations and understand the issue was them

Past experiences often hold us back more than we realise. It can almost feel like our brains are trying to protect us, fearing that what went wrong before is going to happen again.

However, instead of avoiding situations, look at past challenges and ask yourself honestly:

- Was I supported correctly?
- Would the situation have been different if I had got support?
- Was the expectation unreasonable – even for someone without dyslexia?

Reframing past experiences as situations that failed you – rather than your brain failing the situations – is essential for rebuilding confidence. Not only will it stop the situation haunting you, but it will also help you understand the value of getting support and not trying to hide your dyslexia.

Stop making little jokes about your dyslexia

A common strategy among dyslexic people is making jokes about their dyslexic mistakes. I know I did it myself – it felt easier to take control of the situation than to wait for someone else to say something. I instinctively assumed a remark was coming, so I got in first.

Here are a few examples I've heard over the years:

- 'I couldn't organise a piss-up in a brewery.'
- 'I am such a blonde.'
- 'I have a memory like a goldfish.'

But as we've discussed before, hating yourself doesn't help – and neither do these jokes. They hand people the keys to your deepest insecurities. I've had jokes I've made about myself repeated in annual reviews as examples showing where I wasn't capable.

In the workplace, perception is reality. If you make comments about what you can't do, it undermines others' trust in your abilities. Worse, it reinforces your own internal narrative of 'can't' – when the truth is more nuanced.

It's not: 'I can't do this.'

It's: 'I can do it – I just have to do it differently.'

Deal with the negativity of other people

If you've faced negativity around your dyslexia, I'm truly sorry. I know how much it hurts and makes you retreat. But frankly, we need to see it as a 'them' problem.

You're not alone, and you're certainly not unusual. There's a vast number of people who think like you, and what we're asking for – support, understanding, flexibility – isn't unreasonable.

Those who respond with narrow-minded and cruel comments should be ashamed of themselves. And honestly, if they knew even half the truth of our experiences, I believe many would be. The cruellest people are often projecting their own shame on to you!

At this point, you may be thinking: *Natalie, you're asking me to own something proudly that not everyone believes is a strength.*

Here's my take on how to handle that reality:

1. **It is a statement about them, not you**
   As I just said, when someone is being rude or waving red flags, your job isn't to prove yourself – it's to walk away. Their behaviour reflects poor management, a toxic workplace or a lack of understanding of how to change their approach – not your abilities.

2. **It's ignorance, not malice**
   Most of the time, rudeness stems from ignorance, not cruelty. Yes, some people are genuinely cruel, but don't let their opinions affect you. They simply don't understand what you are capable of.

3. **Feel sorry for their lack of strengths**
   This one is a bit cheeky – but once my clients really start recognising their dyslexic strengths, they often feel sad for those who *can't* function or see things the way they do. It's not that they are 'better' than others – it's about recognising that their value is real. It's OK to bring something brilliant to the table and to need support in other areas.

4. **Hating yourself won't help**
   Yes, the mistakes are annoying but building good systems doesn't start with days of self-loathing. It starts with self-respect, strategy and support.

How companies can support sustainable confidence

We all know that a good boss can make or break a workplace – especially for a neurodiverse person. Here are four shifts that can break the cycle of low confidence and unlock meaningful change:

1. **Where a role requires imaginative thought, ask for admin support**

    We often talk about two types of thinkers: 1) imaginative and 2) detail-oriented. Most roles now require a blend – even though few people excel at both. Instead of expecting one person to do it all, we need to build well-rounded teams that support each other's strengths.

    If a role requires imagination, we need to think about how to support that thinking. Don't weigh down creative minds with repetitive admin. Be honest about what the role needs and stop trying to mould people into something they're not.

    I've seen imaginative thinkers stuck in roles that demand rote tasks, simply because employers like the idea of having 'great thinkers' in their team. But these people need to be unshackled and not limited by an unsuitable role.

2. **Don't be boxed into one way of working**

    Dyslexic people are often great at seeing new ways of working. Our big-picture thinking helps us to connect problems and solutions, and our brains crave simplicity and efficiency. But many companies are rigid, locked into policies and processes and unwilling to move and bend. This is to the detriment of that workplace. By opening up to flexibility and allowing a new approach, we all win. The dyslexic person finally feels their brain has value – and that value transforms the department or company.

Too often, we are criticised and pushed into one way of working or thinking. The result? The organisation is never able to access the insights we offer and no one is able to gain.

3. **Let go of what is 'easy'**
   Just because something is easy for you doesn't make it easy for everyone. Labelling tasks as 'easy' when they're not creates shame, not change.

   Instead, have honest conversations about what is genuinely difficult *for you*. This way, we can build better systems and approaches, which will yield more successful results.

4. **Embrace AI**
   There's never been a better time to be dyslexic. The advancement of AI has made managing dyslexic challenges easier than ever before, making support more accessible and allowing strengths to shine.

   Yet many companies restrict the use of AI, unsure how to navigate this change in the way the world works. But AI can do the heavy lifting on tasks that many dyslexic people find difficult – freeing up cognitive space for dyslexic strengths to be unlocked.

Section Two

Unlocking dyslexic strategies

In section 1 we built up an understanding of how to think about dyslexia more confidently and how to let go of a lot of the thoughts and feelings that make building strategies difficult. In this section we are going to take a deep dive into the most common challenges that impact dyslexic people and provide strategies to manage those. The goal is to help you understand your dyslexia better so you can predict when problems are likely to occur. We will also help you build better approaches to managing it.

When looking at building successful dyslexic strategies, it's important to understand there isn't one silver bullet. Instead, we need to use thousands of micro-approaches to different situations.

How to use this section

I hope this section will give you the tools you need – as a reference guide when you have a particular problem, but also as the starting point for building your own strategies. Feel free to read them all in order, to create a clear picture, or follow your gut and dip into the chapters that tackle the challenges you most want to explore – but do read chapters 6 and 7 first, please! Here's what's covered:

- The section opens with an important chapter on how to select which strategies to use and how to get the most out of them, to help you feel less overwhelmed by the many areas dyslexia impacts. Please do take the time to read it, since it will make implementing the advice much easier. And that's where the real work lies: in implementing the strategies in your life.

- Chapter 7 then provides invaluable advice on how to talk about your dyslexia in a constructive way with friends, family and colleagues. A large part of successfully implementing the strategies lies in this communication, so it's important you get it right.

- The rest of the chapters in the section cover the core dyslexic challenges:

Chapter 8: Tiredness

Chapter 9: Working memory

Chapter 10: Interviewing

Chapter 11: Executive functions

Chapter 12: Slow processing

Chapter 13: Reading and writing

Each is examined in turn, first considering why it's a problem, and then providing detailed solutions and strategies that you can put in place. Each chapter ends with information you can pass on to employers, if relevant, so that they can help you achieve your full potential.

6
How to get the most out of the strategies

Chapter summary

Why this chapter is important

Many dyslexic people struggle with understanding which challenges are due to their dyslexia. They might know that they are struggling, but not why. This can make it hard to know which challenge to tackle first. In fact, lots of people end up adopting a scattergun approach and trying to deal with multiple issues at once. Although this appeals to our 'all or nothing' brains and promises great rewards, the truth is that it just makes everything harder. You have to select which challenges you need to work on first and then be methodical. This chapter will help you do that.

What you will learn

- How to identify the areas you need to work on, and which strategies you need.
- What the end goals of the strategies are.
- How you can better implement strategies.
- How companies can better implement strategies.

What strategies do you need?

To help you understand where to start, I recommend you ask yourself two simple questions:

1. What do I find hard?
2. What makes me tired?

Write down everything you can think of, then put your responses in order, from most hard/tiring to least hard/tiring. This should highlight the core areas that you struggle with. You can then arrange these in order of priority for how they *affect your life*. It might not matter that you find checking figures hard, for instance, if you never need to do it, whereas sending an email that doesn't contain inaccurate information is likely a high priority.

As a rule of thumb, I recommend not focusing on more than three problems at a time. The key here is getting comfortable and confident with new approaches and processes before you move on to the next one.

Giving yourself enough time to focus on each new approach and system is essential for driving success.

What is the end goal?

The common messaging to dyslexic people is 'if you do things differently, everything will be OK'. However, to me this has always sounded a bit vague, making it hard to work out your path forwards. So I have created the following metrics to help you understand what you need to do, so you can feel that you have built successful strategies for your dyslexia. Here are the three key elements:

1. To build a toolkit of strategies

The goal is to have strategies that make your brain feel more accessible. All too often, dyslexic challenges can strike and leave us feeling lost about how to deal with them. Instead, we deserve to feel like we have a tried-and-tested list of strategies that work. When I'm describing this, I'm imagining a toolbox that contains a set of trusted hammers, wrenches and other tools that are worn from constant use – because we know they do the job.

Because dyslexia can feel inconsistent, sometimes you feel perfectly capable and sometimes dyslexia comes and trips you up. We need to have day-to-day tools that make mundane moments manageable, as well as power tools for the big moments in life or when dyslexia really shows up.

You may not need to use your toolkit every day, but you deserve to know that when you need them, they are there, ready for when life gets chaotic.

2. To feel capable

Strategies are for more than just helping you not fail: if anything, their most important job is to ensure you *succeed*. Good strategies make you feel like you can:

- Learn that language.
- Go for that promotion.
- Do that project you have secretly thought about for years.

You deserve to do anything you want and not be held back by any fears or dyslexic challenges.

3. To not feel exhausted

Managing dyslexia the hard way – putting in lots of extra hours of hard work without the scaffolding of strategies – can be exhausting.

That not only isn't fair, because it will make the challenges harder, but it also makes life harder to enjoy. It's no fun to come home in the evening so tired that you can't discuss anything and all you can do is watch trash TV.

How do I implement strategies?

Dyslexia can't be perfectly managed, and trying to use strategies every single day can be exhausting and difficult. To help you stay consistent, here are a few pointers to make strategy use more sustainable:

1. Messy action is better than perfectionism

Putting strategies into practice is messy. Often, the desire to implement something perfectly can be a dyslexic person's downfall. I always remind my clients that you are successfully implementing your strategies if you use them 80 per cent of the time or even if you are able to do part of what we have suggested. Remember, something is always better than nothing.

2. Give strategies a chance

Clients often tell me they've already tried things and they didn't work the first time or only worked once we tweaked them. Strategies don't always instantly or completely solve a problem, but they make things easier or less tiring – and that's valuable.

So rather than discarding a strategy because it didn't work once, ask yourself why it didn't work. Here are some useful questions for yourself:

- Did I properly implement the strategy?
- Did the strategy help more than doing nothing?
- What do I want to happen differently that might inform better strategies?

One imperfect result doesn't mean it's not worth continuing.

3. You need to be proactive

Being proactive with strategies is essential. Time and again, I see dyslexic people struggle through a situation until they realise they need to ask for support – often when others have become frustrated with them. Asking for support once a mistake has occurred or after challenges have become significant can be too late or lead to others not being supportive.

Instead, where possible, try to anticipate potential challenges and seek support before they arise. This will help you feel more confident and let others see that you are working hard to do a good job.

4. Acceptance is key

Understanding your challenges and the way your brain works helps you move away from the mindset of *I need to work harder* to *I need strategies or systems to achieve these results*. Accepting that your brain is different – and that your challenges stem from that difference – is essential for driving change.

Personally, I find this concept really valuable. It reminds me to do things differently and to seek out strategies, rather than just piling on shame. But it can feel like a difficult shift, especially when we've spent years believing we just need to try harder. Instead, I like to think: *My brain wasn't built for this, so I need to put in place strategies to make it possible.* Accepting how hard a task is – and how hard it is for *me* – is what helps me lead with strategies and remember to use them consistently.

Without acceptance, I consistently see people finding themselves stuck in a loop of:

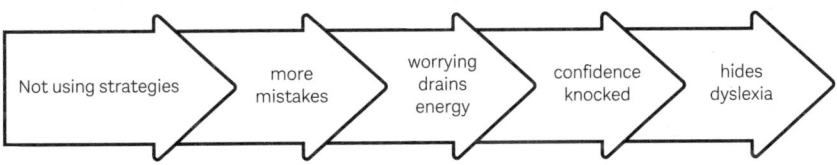

With acceptance, we are able to:

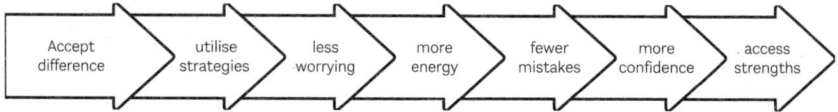

Accept difference → utilise strategies → less worrying → more energy → fewer mistakes → more confidence → access strengths

5. Radical acceptance – not everything needs a strategy

Strategies take time and effort to implement. It's said that a habit takes around 60 repetitions to feel natural. So it's important to be honest about the energy required for us to make changes and embed strategies into daily life.

Sometimes, the most helpful approach to managing dyslexia is to accept minor challenges and let things slip through the net. This isn't about not caring or giving up on being the best version of yourself – it's about choosing where to invest your time and effort and focusing on the areas with the biggest wins.

> **Trying to change every aspect all at once is an almost guaranteed path to failure.**

If you find yourself accidentally adding too many new strategies to your to-do list this week, remember: with my coaching clients, I don't introduce more than three ideas at a time. And if, after a few weeks, we've discussed lots of changes and new ideas, I usually suggest taking a break from coaching to let those ideas settle before adding more.

I also push back if a client brings a problem that seems like it'll take a lot of work to change but might not make a big impact. In those cases, my first suggestion is usually: 'Let's think about acceptance first.'

How companies can support strategies

At work, it can be nerve-wrecking to stand up and admit that you need support. To make things easier, for each of the remaining chapters in this section I'm going to give you some pointers that will help you ask for what you need. If you're reading this as an employer, these are the proactive things you can do to help your dyslexic staff feel confident and capable.

1. Remember that these strategies benefit everyone

As I constantly remind my clients: what works best for dyslexic people will also likely work well for everyone else. These aren't just strategies and ways of working that solely benefit individuals; they will make your entire team more productive and able to manage tasks more effectively.

So instead of seeing these policies as bespoke to accommodate an individual, why not implement them as standard?

2. Staff are legally entitled to reasonable adjustments

In the UK, and many other countries, the law is very clear that reasonable adjustments should be made to support dyslexic employees. What counts as 'reasonable' is more than most employers and even employees realise, so you need to do your research. I think a lot of the challenges and frustrations would be minimised if companies really understood the truth of their responsibilities.

3. Stop shaming staff for being dyslexic

I have made a deliberate effort to talk about the emotional experience of being dyslexic, sharing the reality of how every dyslexic person I speak to is already trying their best to manage their challenges. Often, they feel more mortified by their struggles than any manager or colleague ever could.

It's important to reframe the conversation around neurodiversity: assume that hard work and effort are already happening, and avoid trying to drive change through shame. In my life – and in the thousands of conversations I've had with dyslexic individuals – the pattern is clear: if we could have changed already, we would have.

Change doesn't come from shame. It comes from strategies.

7

How to talk about dyslexia with others

Chapter summary

Why this chapter is important

In section 1, we explored how understanding your own dyslexia is essential for rebuilding confidence and laying solid foundations. Once those foundations are in place, strategies can be set on top.

This section focuses on the core strategies you need to manage dyslexia successfully. As you begin to apply these strategies, you'll likely find yourself needing to explain to others how you work and manage being neurodiverse.

That's why this feels like the right moment to discuss how to handle those conversations – successfully and with confidence.

What you will learn

- How and when to discuss dyslexia at work.
- How to discuss dyslexia in your personal life.

When we talk about managing dyslexia and navigating conversations around it, the frameworks I've developed are designed to flex with individual circumstances, legal situations, cultural norms and personal experiences.

The most important thing is to try to approach these conversations with confidence. If you feel comfortable talking about dyslexia and sharing that proudly – fantastic. But if you don't, there are still simple strategies you can use to discuss your needs without ever mentioning the word 'dyslexia'.

How to discuss dyslexia at work

Here's a straightforward framework for when, where and how to talk about dyslexia in the workplace:

1. When to discuss dyslexia

I believe it's best to raise dyslexia as early as possible. This gives you the chance to talk about accommodations and strengths in a neutral setting, before any challenges arise.

> **Early disclosure allows you to control the narrative and set yourself up for success.**

If you wait too long, dyslexia may only come up in response to a difficulty or mistake – which can frame the conversation negatively and make it harder to build trust. When dyslexia is tied to a problem, it's easy for others to see it as the cause, especially if strategies haven't already been put in place.

Here are some key moments when you might choose to discuss dyslexia, with pros and cons for each:

At interview

Pros: This allows you to discuss dyslexia and clarify whether the role is a good fit for your strengths and support needs.

Cons: It can feel daunting and requires confidence. You'll need to be clear on your strengths and what support you need – something many people are still working on.

Just after receiving a job offer

Pros: This is a common and safe moment to disclose, especially in the UK, where withdrawing an offer would likely be unlawful. You can have a fair and frank conversation before leaving your current role.

Cons: It may feel awkward to share such an important fact that you didn't raise at interview. You'll need clarity on your strategies and strengths, as you'll likely be asked, 'How can I support you?'

When you first start the job

Pros: People expect new starters to have unique strengths and challenges. It's a natural time to make accommodations or changes to processes.

Cons: You may not yet understand the role well enough to explain clearly what will work for you.

A year into the job

Pros: You'll have a clear sense of the role and what might work better. It's never too late to make changes and improvements.

Cons: If you didn't have support at the beginning, you may have had a bumpy start and it might be harder to reframe the conversation positively.

Straight after reading this book

Pros: The knowledge you have gained can spark a conversation and help you feel confident about discussing dyslexia.

Cons: None! If you're not yet confident, you can use strategies that don't require naming dyslexia directly – *see* p. 109.

2. Where to discuss dyslexia

It's crucial to discuss dyslexia confidently and in a way that both builds trust and makes it clear you are capable. This is why my key piece of advice is to avoid linking dyslexia disclosure to a recent mistake. Instead, aim for a neutral moment and location when you can explain your strategies and strengths clearly.

Ideally, have the conversation in a private meeting where you can break down the support you need and demonstrate what you can bring to the role. Avoid casual mentions over the desk or disclosures made in the heat of a problem – these rarely allow for the full, constructive conversation that's needed.

3. How to discuss dyslexia for the first time

Here's my tried-and-tested formula for a successful dyslexia conversation:

Step one: Explain dyslexia.

Step two: Share the strategies or support you use or need.

Step three: Reaffirm your capability and track record.

Step four: Highlight your strengths with examples.

Example script:

Hello Lauren,

> I wanted to talk to you about my dyslexia. I'm not sure how much you know about it, but it affects how I process information and means I approach certain tasks differently. This brings some challenges – and also some great opportunities.

A few tasks I find difficult are:

- Checking important documents alone
- Processing large amounts of information in a short time frame
- Managing multiple priorities at once

Some strategies that work well for me are:

- Allowing time for a second pair of eyes on key documents.
- Starting with an overview when receiving new information, and repeating key points.
- Including a priorities check-in during our weekly one-to-ones.

I know dyslexia isn't always well understood, but I have managed it successfully throughout my education and in every workplace so far. I feel confident that with a few small adjustments, this will be no different.

Being dyslexic and processing things differently gives me strengths I'm proud of and keen to use in my role. These include:

- I find that ideas come easily to me and I enjoy understanding a topic and coming up with new ways of approaching a problem.
- I connect well with people and really enjoy making presentations engaging and persuasive.

4. How to discuss ad hoc dyslexic challenges confidently

If you need to raise a specific issue or request support, here's a simple approach – whether or not you mention dyslexia:

Ask early – Asking for support in advance shows that you're proactive and organised.

Be specific – Most people don't understand dyslexia and won't know how to help unless you're clear.

Show how it helps them – People are naturally focused on outcomes. Frame your request in terms of what it enables you to achieve. Here's an example script:

> For the upcoming project, could we arrange weekly 15-minute catch-ups to review progress and discuss any questions? I find this helps me meet deadlines and resolve issues quickly.

Tip: notice I didn't discuss dyslexia at all. If you want to say, 'because I am dyslexic', that is great if you feel it will add weight to your request, but it isn't always necessary. The goal is to help others see how the support helps you do your best.

Here's what people often do instead – which isn't helpful:

> 'Sorry to bother you. I know it's a bit annoying, but would you mind helping me with the new project? I really struggle with staying on task and managing deadlines, so I would really appreciate a weekly catch-up to help me stay focused.'

You can understand why people feel nervous asking for support – especially when it's framed in such a negative way. Focusing on what support helps you achieve is a much more confident and effective way to talk about dyslexia.

5. Who should you tell?

This is a tricky one to answer, as so much depends on the context. Here are some prompts to help you decide:

Do I trust this person not to judge me? – Unfortunately, many people have preconceptions about dyslexia. Disclosure can carry risks, so trust is key.

Will I get meaningful support by saying something? – Not everyone needs to know. Sometimes, sharing can feel like making an 'excuse' when really it's just about doing things differently. That's why our approach – 'this will help me do my best' – can be so effective.

Do I feel confident enough to discuss dyslexia? – If you don't feel confident, you may over-focus on the challenges and undersell your strengths. It's OK to wait until you feel ready to have the conversation in a way that reflects your capability.

Discussing dyslexia in your personal life

In a funny way, talking about dyslexia at work can sometimes feel simpler. There's a clearer path, a kind of dance that's been done before – a formula you can follow, even if it's awkward or scary. But updating friends, family and partners about your neurodiversity can feel uncomfortable and odd, especially when they feel like they already 'know' you.

As I said in the introduction, I was diagnosed with dyslexia when I was seven but only realised I had ADHD in my late twenties – a common experience for women. So my lateness, constant misplacing of things, general disorganisation and distractedness were seen as 'character defects', not symptoms. I worked hard to mask these traits. But when I started building a life that worked better with my ADHD, I let the mask down and started being myself.

It was my personal life that took the most adjustment. People had known me pre-diagnosis, and now I was asking for support, expecting kindness and no longer putting myself second just to appear 'normal'. That shift – unmasking and asking for what I needed – was the hardest for those closest to me to understand.

So when it comes to explaining neurodiversity to a generation unfamiliar with it, or to people who knew you before diagnosis, it can be hard. I know – I've been in the trenches! Here are my tips on how to make that transition easier:

1. Share resources

Try not to take it personally, but sometimes it's easier for people to learn from a neutral, or ideally official, source. Sharing articles, videos or books about neurodiversity is a great way to reinforce what you're trying to explain and gives your loved ones a broader understanding.

2. Ask for kindness

Kindness goes a long way. Shame is often the tool that is used to push change, especially around neurodiversity – passive-aggressive reminders, little jokes about past mistakes, or a lack of trust over simple tasks. These chip away at your confidence, entrench shame and do nothing to build systems that work.

When you're asking for kindness, you're asking people to see your challenges as symptoms not as character flaws and to help you have the space to create solutions rather than pressure to conform. Frankly, if the pressure worked, you wouldn't be needing the diagnosis in the first place!

> **How I explain it to those who are close to me is: I can't always live life with a system. Sometimes I need to relax. I can't spend every moment constantly thinking about the next task or process. When something isn't important, I need slack – not a lecture.**

Here are some examples of what kindness looks like:

- Explaining card games twice without sighs or comments.
- Not getting annoyed when you forgot the item you went to the shops for.
- Listening and reassuring when reading aloud is bumpy.
- Gently reminding you of important appointments.
- Not reacting when you say 'left' but mean 'right'.
- Staying calm during public transport muddles.
- Helping talk through household task timings to see what's reasonable.
- Sending the name of the restaurant in advance so you can read the menu without pressure.
- Putting subtitles on films as standard.
- Not pointing out 'your' v 'you're' errors – because they understand what you meant.

3. It takes time

Changing your perception of someone and understanding neurodiversity takes time. People don't always grasp it straight away, but that's OK. Neurodiversity is unpredictable. You'll have 'good periods' and 'challenging eras'. Seeing both sides of the coin – and witnessing the effort that still results in failure – is key to recognising that these challenges aren't within your control.

Time helps people see that these traits are consistent and real. It also helps them grow accustomed to the unmasked, newly understood version of you.

4. Your own self-acceptance is most important

If people in your life don't understand neurodiversity as quickly as you would like, it's OK to focus on your own self-acceptance. Keep building your strategies. Keep practising kindness towards yourself. Let others catch up in their own time.

8
Tiredness

> **Chapter summary**
>
> **Why this chapter is important**
>
> The exhaustion you experience due to dyslexia is no joke – it's one of the most significant challenges facing all neurodiverse people. It can range from feeling like you can't do any more in the afternoon because your brain is broken with tiredness, to having multiple cycles of burnout. Either way, its impact is significant.
>
> Asking our brains to repeatedly do things we find difficult uses a lot of energy. Yet this aspect of dyslexia is often not openly discussed, which means people don't understand what is going on and don't build the correct solutions.
>
> I remember finishing work most evenings so brain-dead all I could do was watch TV and go to bed early, unable to have a conversation or even watch a complex TV show. Sadly, this is the reality for many dyslexic people: they feel numb in the evening and unable to enjoy their leisure time, or worry about how to keep going because they have hit burnout. But it shouldn't be like this. This chapter is all about providing you with strategies to manage fatigue and reduce its impact.

> **What you will learn**
> - The daily reality of dyslexia and exhaustion.
> - The significant impact burnout has on our community.
> - Steps you can take to better manage daily tiredness.
> - How to break the cycle of dyslexia and burnout.

Understanding why tiredness is a problem

Of all the problems I discuss with dyslexic individuals, exhaustion crops up most frequently. In fact, the videos I've created on this topic are among our most watched and downloaded.

There are several reasons why you might be struggling with tiredness right now:

- Difficulty saying no, meaning you overstretch yourself.
- The neurological make-up of your brain.
- Not taking sufficient breaks.
- Working too hard to compensate for dyslexic challenges.

Below, we'll explore each of these in turn – then move on to practical strategies you can use to manage and reduce fatigue.

1. Low confidence means you find it hard to say no

Confidence plays a leading role in the exhaustion many of us face – and it's a key contributor to the cycles of burnout that dyslexic people often find themselves in. For many, confidence has been shredded by years of negative feedback, leading to a fear of communicating needs or pushing back. There's a deep worry that saying no will make others think we're not up to the job or task.

Over and over again I see dyslexic people stretching themselves too thin – saying yes to everything to prove how capable they are. This then leads to working late or overcommitting to non-work activities, sacrificing weekends trying to manage an impossible workload.

> ## Real-world story
>
> One woman came to me as a coaching client after multiple cycles of burnout and periods of sick leave. She was anxious that her fast-paced, ideas-centric workplace would push her to overextend herself – something she was already doing in every other area of her life, from friendships to family to church.
>
> She arrived with a bag full of strategies, confused about why she was still in the office until 8 p.m. with a long list of tasks due the next day. She had no visibility of her workload and no system to manage it, so she kept saying yes and piling on more.
>
> Together, we worked on building awareness of her workload and acknowledging that by constantly saying yes, she was in fact doing her company a disservice. We explored how she could push back, say no, set boundaries and protect her time so that she could show up consistently and meet deadlines with greater ease and fewer mistakes. Once she had more consistent energy, she could focus on what worked, without needing long periods of sick leave every few years to recover.
>
> Seeing everything she was doing – and having a clearer picture of the value she was providing – helped her shift from constantly proving herself, to saying no and doing less, better.

2. Brain make-up makes tasks harder

Much of modern life is made up of tasks that dyslexic brains don't naturally find easy. That means we have to work harder to achieve the same results. Whether it's reading messages, checking train times or processing instructions, these seemingly simple tasks require extra focus and effort.

The neuroscience is clear: dyslexic people typically show reduced activity in the left hemisphere of the brain, which handles language and reading. This means we are constantly having to push our brains to do things that are inherently more difficult for us – which builds up exhaustion over the day.

When we don't acknowledge that certain tasks take more out of us, we fail to plan our day effectively.

For example, reading a recipe might require more focus than expected, and if we don't allow enough time or breaks, it takes longer than expected and we end up rushing into the next task and feeling drained.

> ### Real-world story
>
> As I write this, my cheeks are red because I am reliving the embarrassment all over again.
>
> Before I understood how to manage dyslexia, the 3 p.m. wall of tiredness was a daily battle for me. It felt like my brain had an off-switch. Once I hit that point, I was done. I used to visualise it as a thick fog descending over my mind. Once it settled, no new information could get in or out.
>
> One afternoon, after a string of long meetings and intense processing, I had to write a detailed email summarising the decisions. My brain felt like it had run a marathon doing everything it liked least. The brain fog was thick. I tried a third coffee, but nothing could revive me.
>
> Ideally, I should've accepted that the day was done and saved the workload for tomorrow. Instead, I filled the time with light tasks – or let's be honest, pretended to work.
>
> That day, I ended up watching YouTube videos for about 20 minutes. During that time, the senior director of my department

> tapped me on the shoulder with an urgent question – and saw the video. 'Are you watching YouTube instead of working?' he asked.
>
> I wanted the ground to swallow me whole. It's not like I could turn around and say, 'Sorry, I'm dyslexic and tired and can't work for the next two hours.' But that was the truth – bad systems, no breaks and no understanding of how my brain worked meant I was completely spent.

3. You don't take sufficient breaks

Many dyslexic people feel that their way of working or their needs aren't 'acceptable' in modern workplaces – or modern life in general. Because some tasks take longer, we often feel the need to 'make up' for it by skipping breaks and working through.

But skipping breaks doesn't help. It reduces processing speed, increases the likelihood of mistakes, and makes everything more inefficient.

Often, people avoid breaks for hours – or the whole day – because they feel behind. Then they crash at the end of the day. One of the saddest patterns I hear regularly is people avoiding holidays altogether because they feel perpetually behind.

4. You use working hard as a strategy

Hard work is the childhood best friend of many dyslexic people. From a young age, we learned that success meant putting in extra hours and extra effort. And many of us have continued to rely on that strategy into adult life.

What that means is that we are comfortable with hard work, wherever that crops up. It feels normal to put in more hours to achieve the same results. But this over-reliance on effort – and underuse of strategies –

means we're often wading through quicksand. Burnout creeps in and we don't always recognise it.

The result? We accept bad situations. We expect a lack of support. And we heap the responsibility on ourselves. This leads to higher rates of burnout in our community and makes it harder to advocate for realistic, supportive changes.

> **Real-world story**
>
> At school, I used to really struggle with getting the same grades as my peers and often felt like I wasn't living up to my potential. I found that the best way for me to improve was to redo any of my exams or homework that hadn't gone well, to try to get better grades the second time (I am aware of how much of a teacher's pet I was!). It worked: I'd start with a B, take the feedback and redo the work to get an A. It was here that hard work was drilled into me.
>
> I remember someone at work once saying to me they were surprised at how much I went above and beyond to get things done. I told them that it was nothing compared to how I used to behave at school.

Strategies for tiredness

Now that we've explored the reasons why dyslexia can be so exhausting, you can begin to proactively spot patterns, avoid common pitfalls and identify areas you want to improve. Below are the core strategies I regularly share with my clients to help them feel more consistent in their energy levels – so they're not permanently exhausted or one step away from a cycle of burnout.

These strategies are designed to make everyday tasks easier to manage, reduce cognitive load, and help you build structure around breaks and energy management.

Strategy one: the 80:20 rule

The 80:20 rule helps you build a framework for thinking about support – whether that's a friend reviewing your CV or a manager spellchecking your important work. It helps you stop working at 200 per cent while still honouring the dyslexic value of hard work. Because if it were as simple as 'just work less', you'd be doing it already. This strategy channels your hard-working tendencies into a more sustainable, productive system.

What is the 80:20 rule?

You take on 80 per cent of the workload and responsibility, while allowing others to support you with the remaining 20 per cent, either by helping you with tasks you find harder or allowing them to be done differently. Essentially, it's a practical way to think about 'reasonable adjustments'.

The 80:20 rule in everyday life: going to the supermarket

You're doing 80 per cent of the work:

- Getting to the supermarket.
- Going around and picking the items.
- Returning home.
- Putting the food away.

20 per cent support could include:

- Helping you plan what food is needed.
- Texting you the list so you don't rely on working memory.
- Providing accountability for tedious tasks like unpacking.

What 200 per cent used to look like:

- Writing half the list and assuming you would remember the rest – then having to go back for forgotten items.
- Being reminded the next day you forgot something else, and having to wake up early to go again.
- Losing sleep and spending time going back and forwards, and feeling mad at yourself for the oversight.

The 80:20 rule in work life: report writing
You're doing 80 per cent of the work:

- Gathering information.
- Ordering and mapping out the flow of the document.
- Writing the first draft.
- Ensuring the document meets the needs of the end user.

20 per cent support could include:

- Collaborative brain-dump sessions to break down ideas and reduce procrastination.
- Mini deadlines and check-ins to ensure work is done regularly and not all near the deadline.
- Where possible, providing templates to help you visualise the report's structure.
- Reviewing the document for typos and phrasing.
- Allowing AI to organise thoughts and check the document.

What 200 per cent used to look like:

- Not getting support with getting started, leading to procrastination and embarrassment, and the need to rush.
- Not getting help to organise your ideas, meaning you started the report without a plan, making it harder to edit.
- Not getting help with spellchecking the document, meaning you had to take it home to read multiple times to find every tiny mistake – turning a 30-minute task into a two-hour ordeal.

Even small adjustments like these – where you still do the bulk of the work – can significantly reduce exhaustion.

The key is remembering that asking for support doesn't mean doing less – it means doing it smarter.

Working at 200 per cent might feel like the easier option in the short term, but in the long run, it's not serving you – or those around you.

Strategy two: managing your capacity

Saying no can feel terrifying. You might worry people will think you're slow or incapable. But allowing tasks to just pile up without a clear plan isn't a solution either. It might feel easier in the moment to say yes, but it often leads to missed deadlines.

Here's the solution: slow down decision-making. Give yourself time to process requests and make a plan.

For many dyslexic people, low confidence and slower processing make it tempting to say yes immediately. Instead, get comfortable with making decisions later – once you have had a chance to assess your workload or what else is going on in your life. Here are some example responses to help you:

- I want to make sure I can give this the time it deserves. Can I confirm with you by [time frame]?
- I don't want to rush my response – can I take a little time to think it through and let you know?
- This is important to me, so I want to make sure I can do it properly. I'll get back to you by [time frame].
- I don't want to overpromise, so I need to take a step back and check what's realistic. I'll get back to you soon.

The reframe

It can be easy to think *I'm incapable* but actually it's about managing your workload and energy efficiently and effectively. Saying yes too quickly might feel helpful, but it often leads to bigger problems later. Hard conversations are easier – and more productive – when they happen early.

Strategy three: take brain breaks

As dyslexics, we know we need to take more regular brain breaks. But knowing what is best for you and actually doing it are two different things. In this section I want to share how to approach breaks and build them more seamlessly into your life.

Step one is shifting your mindset from *I don't have time to take breaks* to *I need to take breaks to stay productive*. Learning how long your brain can work before needing a reset is essential.

I find that scheduling breaks is the only way I can actually make them happen.

Here are some other tips:

1. Know what you need

I know I can't work past 8 p.m. – my brain starts to turn to mush. With clients in the USA, that's tricky, but honouring my limits helps me show up at my best.

2. Factor in rest

When I book meetings, I build in gaps of 15–30 minutes. I've accepted that these aren't for squeezing in extra tasks – they're for resetting my brain and allowing me to keep going.

3. Set expectations ahead of time

You might not realise you need a break until it's too late. Scheduling breaks in your diary – or setting a minimum number per day – helps you take action before burnout hits.

4. Plan natural breaks

Stopping between tasks can feel really frustrating. So finish a task, take five minutes to walk around, then dive into the next chunk.

5. Little breaks, not long ones

We all know we should do this – and yet we don't. Clients often keep pushing with no breaks until they feel brain-dead, then need longer breaks to recover. As a rule of thumb, I suggest that every two hours you get up and walk around for five minutes. It makes a huge difference.

> ### Real-world story
>
> At a recent conference, I spoke to someone about energy management. Her main complaint was that she felt like she needed hours to recharge and rest and that her brain was letting her down. She wanted to work on a side hustle but didn't have the energy to manage working, having a life and building a passion project.
>
> After a little bit of digging, I realised she wasn't taking any breaks at all during the day. She was getting frustrated that she then needed to sleep all weekend.
>
> When I encouraged her to take breaks, she told me she didn't have time. I tried to make the argument that it would benefit her in the long run, since she would gain back the time in improved productivity.
>
> We continued in this way for a few minutes, with her forcefully pushing back, until I finally asked her to explain why breaks felt so impossible. Her answer was: 'I don't have an hour a day to take breaks.' I told her: 'Neither do I. I just take 15 minutes every few hours.' And if she did too, she would likely see huge improvements in her energy levels.

What are brain breaks?

When we keep pushing, our brains naturally begin to slow down and we find ourselves taking breaks without even realising – accidentally spending too long on our phones or staring into space. But when we don't fully accept the need for a break, and instead try to force ourselves back into focus, those moments don't feel restful. They don't reset us – which can mean work slows down.

Try reframing breaks as part of your productivity strategy. They're not interruptions; they're essential tools that help you keep going at the speed you want. Instead of fighting breaks, make them part of the plan.

Here are some I recommend and one I don't:

1. **Something physical**
   A walk or simply getting up from your desk gives your mind the reset it needs.
   Rating: 9/10 – even something small can be mighty.
2. **Naps**
   Naps can be a dyslexic person's best friend and really help prepare your mind for a new task – perfect if you're able to work from home.
   Rating: 10/10 – it's a shame it isn't more socially acceptable at work.
3. **Doing something you enjoy**
   Engaging in something you're good at and enjoy can light you up and activate different parts of the brain.
   Rating: 7/10 – helpful, but it can be tiring if your brain's already fatigued.
4. **Scrolling on your phone**
   It's common (guilty here, too), but it still demands significant processing power and rarely gives your brain the break it needs.
   Rating: 2/10 – still cognitively demanding, even if it feels passive.

Strategy four: re-evaluate what is easy

One of the big mistakes dyslexic people make is using neurotypical standards to judge what is 'easy' and what is 'hard'. By redefining what *you* find easy, it becomes more obvious when you need a break or when you've overexerted yourself.

Many clients push through tasks they assume are easy, believing they 'should' be able to keep going. But by recognising your own version of 'easy', you can build a better relationship with energy management.

Here are a few examples of dyslexic challenges that may seem simple but can be cognitively draining for dyslexic brains:

1. Listening and focusing for extended periods (such as listening to a speaker at a conference or focusing in a meeting).
2. Planning any type of public transport journey.
3. Completing forms and paperwork.

Even if these tasks seem minor, they may require a break afterwards.

How companies can support strategies for tiredness

Today's work culture often champions productivity and sees the workforce as a company's core asset. Here are some ways organisations can support their dyslexic employees in managing the energy demands of neurodiversity, to help them be more productive, reduce mistakes and increase access to strengths:

1. Review flexible hours and working from home (WFH) policies

We're adults at work and should be treated as such. This means allowing staff to work in ways and at times that best support their productivity. For instance:

- Dyslexic individuals may prefer working more in the mornings and leaving earlier, since cognitive fatigue builds throughout the day.
- People with ADHD may have different circadian rhythms and work better later in the day.

Policies should centre on productivity and well-being – not rigid enforcement across the board. Flexibility allows for better energy management and more sustainable performance.

2. Create decompression spaces

Offices need spaces that support focus and decompression. These allow people to take proper breaks – not fake ones where they're still 'on'.

3. Allow roles to evolve

Companies often reserve role evolution for senior members of staff, but dyslexic brains naturally possess many of the most sought-after skills – creativity, problem-solving and big-picture thinking. Yet we're asked to prove ourselves in tasks we find inherently difficult. This keeps us stuck.

Allowing roles to evolve around strengths – and providing support where needed – will help you access the amazing opportunities dyslexic employees bring to the table.

9
Working memory

> **Chapter summary**
>
> **Why this chapter is important**
>
> If you take only one thing away from this book, I want it to be this: how to manage working memory.
>
> Working memory is one of the biggest challenges dyslexic people face – and it's often the hidden reason behind the feeling that 'dyslexia is so much more than issues with reading and writing'.
>
> Most dyslexic individuals struggle with their working memory without realising that's what the problem is. It is by far the biggest issue I see most often in my work. The good news is, it's also the area where we have the most practical, effective strategies to help.
>
> **What you will learn**
> - Why working memory is at the root of many of your challenges.
> - How to understand and explain working memory simply to those around you.

- How to anticipate working memory challenges and prepare proactively.
- Strategies and approaches to managing working memory challenges more effectively.

Understanding working memory

Working memory is the part of the brain that temporarily stores information while it's being processed. It acts like a mental notepad, holding short-term details until they can be transferred into longer-term memory or used to complete a task.

Everyone (not just neurodiverse people) has a limited working memory capacity. On average, most people can hold around six or seven items at once. For dyslexic people, that number tends to be smaller – typically around four or five items.

Let me give you an example. Imagine someone gives you directions to the loo. You remember the first two steps, but then everything else becomes a blur. That's your working memory reaching its limit. It held the first part but couldn't retain the rest.

One of the most important things to understand about working memory is how much it's impacted by stress and tiredness. When you're stressed or fatigued, your capacity is reduced.

So if you find the meetings you have with your close office friend go amazingly – you're clear and articulate – but meetings with a senior manager leave you flustered, talking in circles and being a bit of a blur, it's not just nerves. It's the reality of working memory under pressure.

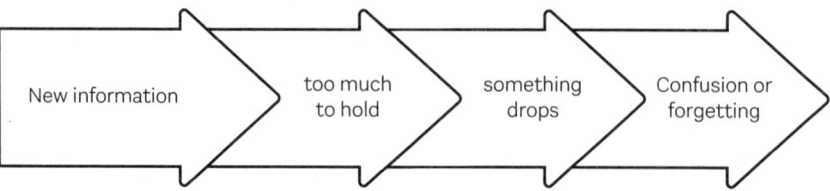

How working memory impacts you

Working memory challenges show up in everyday life in ways that are often frustrating, public and misunderstood. Below are seven key areas where working memory can impact dyslexic individuals, and real-world stories that show how relatable and common they are:

> ### Real-world story
>
> We all know the NHS is under pressure, and occasionally I wince when I read about the cost of missed appointments. Last year, I was trying to get a diagnosis for a chronic condition. After months of waiting, I finally got a referral to a specialist – only to write down the wrong date. So despite the ten alarms and constant reminders, I missed the appointment because I was a day out. Missing the appointment was embarrassing enough, but calling the reception team to explain the situation was mortifying. I went to the back of the queue and had to tell friends and family that I'd messed up again – even though I thought I'd done everything right.

1. Lists of information

This is one of the most obvious – and familiar – working memory challenges. If I listed five numbers and asked you to recall them immediately, you might only remember the first and last.

Because this challenge is something a lot of dyslexics struggle with, it often carries a lot of stress and worry. When someone starts explaining something, our brains can panic – ironically reducing our working memory capacity even further.

Here are a few everyday examples that can feel embarrassing:

- Calling the doctor and writing the appointment date down wrong.
- Typing a new password and then instantly forgetting it.
- When someone verbally explains a process or system and you leave feeling like you just went on a roller coaster.

2. Processing in meetings

Meetings are one of the biggest working memory challenges I support clients with. New information is pummelled at you, often across multiple projects, at a fast pace. This can make it hard to process the information deeply and clearly. This problem overlaps with slow processing, making the challenge even more significant.

Many people leave meetings feeling exhausted from having to concentrate so much, or perhaps having been unable to fully participate or unsure what happened. You might also have lost track of key points or struggled to identify them in the first place. This confusion can lead to disengagement, missed contributions and a cycle of self-doubt.

> ### Real-world story
>
> One client started in the post room and worked his way up over 20 years to become a senior account manager, leading major clients and mentoring some of the junior staff. At school, his teachers had told him he would never achieve anything, but the classic dyslexic combination of hard work, determination, good ideas and an ability to connect with people helped him build a successful career.
>
> But inside, he remembered what his teachers had said, and he carried a large dollop of imposter syndrome. And that was being fed by the difficulties he faced in some meetings.

In small meetings with his team or friendly clients, he felt in control and capable, able to recall information and add value to points raised. But in large meetings – especially those run by the implementation team – everything felt confused and difficult to follow. Problems would arise, multiple solutions would be kicked around, and new pieces of information would flood in. He felt lost, so he stayed quiet as much as possible, hoping nobody would notice.

But his boss did.

My client knew dyslexia was part of the problem but he hadn't heard of working memory. He didn't realise how stress was making it worse, or how lack of clarity and structure in meetings was putting extra pressure on his brain.

All of this had built up over time to the point where on our first call, the first words he said were, 'I'm not sure I can do this job.' I knew he was too determined and resilient and had worked too hard to throw in the towel – but it was hard to hear how much dyslexia was impacting his confidence. The large meetings had left him feeling stupid and embarrassed, so frustrated that even though he was working hard, the problem wasn't going away.

Once my client understood working memory he instantly could see how it was impacting him and how he wasn't useless, he just needed some systems to help him.

So we created structure around these bigger meetings (see 'Strategy two: get the big picture' on p. 140), which helped him follow the flow of information more easily and feel capable in how his brain worked.

3. Word recall

Working memory challenges are often public – and word recall is one of the most common. Like everything else to do with working memory, it tends to worsen with stress or exhaustion.

When your working memory is overloaded, your ability to recall information, including words, is impacted. One of the most frustrating parts is that often you're let down mid-sentence. You're left with three options:

I. Reformat the sentence entirely.
II. Wait in silence, hoping the word returns (it rarely does, because the longer you wait, the more stressed you become).
III. Find a substitute word to fill the gap.

> **Real-world story**
>
> A friend once forgot the word for 'phone' and, in a panic, said 'calling device'. We both knew what he meant – and had a good laugh.

4. Remembering names

Names are my personal nemesis. If more than one person introduces themselves, I don't even try to remember. I focus on other facts about them, and give people pet names to mask the truth that I rarely retain their real ones.

> **Real-world story**
>
> As a coach, I learn about people's lives – their partners, bosses and close friends, either those who are a great help or ones who make their days a misery.

> This means I often need to refer to these characters: 'What did Lucy say?' or 'How did Ben react to that?' But with at least five clients at once, each with their own cast of characters, I can't remember all the names. I usually just guess, hoping for the best. I've worked with one client for two years, and I still try a new name every time for her boyfriend and now-husband. We laugh about it, but it's a real challenge.

5. Communicating ideas clearly

Explaining your thoughts as a dyslexic person can feel embarrassing – like you're talking in circles or sound like a total idiot. This is incredibly frustrating but it does come from a strength.

Dyslexic people often have great ideas. We are complex thinkers who connect multiple ideas quickly and find solutions drop into our minds fully formed. That's a gift – but it comes at a cost.

Our working memory quickly gets overwhelmed when we try to simplify and communicate these ideas – especially when inspiration strikes in the moment and we haven't had the chance to prepare. So you start excitedly sharing your idea but then notice people staring at you, confused. You feel like you have gone around in circles without ever really landing the point.

6. Losing your train of thought

Is there anything worse than losing your train of thought? One moment it's there – important, clear – and the next, it's gone. That's working memory at play again.

A related example: walking into a room or opening the fridge with no idea why you're there or what you wanted. Your thoughts moved on, and your working memory dropped what it was holding.

> **Real-world story**
>
> A few years ago, I had a coaching client who was known for her quick thinking. As soon as a new problem was raised in her team, she could always offer a good solution. She knew her ideas weren't always fully formed, but after years in the role, she felt comfortable being herself and sharing concepts freely.
>
> One day a new senior member joined a meeting. My client's old habits were hard to break, and halfway through explaining an idea she realised she had lost the room; she was talking in circles and then, mid-sentence, she just stopped speaking. The fear and embarrassment had taken hold and in that moment of low confidence it seemed better to abruptly stop than try to wrap up her point.

7. Answering questions

When working memory is under stress, even simple moments can feel like completing an Ironman. Someone asks you a question, especially a long one, and even if you know the answer, stress kicks in and overloads your brain.

Suddenly, a project update you've been working on all week and understand inside out or your own phone number are impossible to recall. That spike in stress shrinks your working memory capacity and leaves you flustered.

Feeling like you can't rely on your brain can lead to self-doubt and that you shouldn't put yourself in positions where things could go wrong. This avoidance keeps people smaller than their brains are capable of – because of fear, not ability.

> ### Real-world story
>
> At a company training session, I spoke with a woman who was upset about the challenges she was having at work. I asked her what her role was, hoping to understand more. She couldn't remember. The stress of the moment had overwhelmed her working memory. She stared at me for what felt like two minutes (but was probably only 10 seconds) saying 'umm' until the stress went away and her ability to process came back. Only then could she explain her job title and her responsibilities.
>
> This is what stress does – and it can really impact your confidence, making the problem even worse.

Strategies for working memory

Managing working memory is essential. As you've seen, it can cause frustration, embarrassment and confusion when you don't know what's going on or how to manage it.

The key is to avoid overloading your working memory. Offload information elsewhere – onto paper, into systems or verbally – so your brain has space to process and remember what matters.

The waiter analogy

Working memory is like a waiter carrying too many plates. If you keep piling them on, eventually they'll fall. The plates end up on the floor and will be forgotten – just like the overloaded information in your brain.

Instead, imagine the waiter carrying only what they can manage. That's how working memory works best: take one or two plates at a time.

> So next time you're feeling overloaded and unable to move forwards, think to yourself: *What can I put down to keep moving forwards?* It's not that you 'can't' process information, you just need a better approach.

Strategy one: control the conversation

When too much information comes at once, your brain drops it – like that waiter with too many plates. You leave the conversation feeling like you have been spun around a hundred times and are left trying to pick up the fragments of information you do remember. Or worse, you're asked a question and realise you don't fully understand everything that was said and are not able to deliver an answer successfully.

Controlling the conversation helps you slow the pace and manage the flow of information. It's one of the most important skills I teach my clients, and applies to all sorts of situations.

What controlling the conversation looks like:

- Don't let someone talk for five minutes straight. Ask them to pause so you can digest what is being said.
- Don't pretend to understand – ask for clarity.
- Use the techniques below to offload information, to help you process everything.

What that sounds like in practice:

- 'Before you go any further, can I repeat what I just heard?'
- 'That's a lot of information – let me grab a pen and paper to ensure I follow everything.'
- 'That all sounds really interesting but we covered a lot. Could you repeat from [point XYZ] so I can get my head around the detail?'

How to break the habit of staying silent

Learning to control the conversation is especially important in scenarios when recording isn't possible or where you need to be able to engage in real time rather than digesting the information after the fact. In these situations, we often choose to stay quiet and hope people don't notice we haven't followed everything.

It's really important to try to break this habit. Speaking up early is better than staying quiet and struggling later and not being able to answer a question successfully. You deserve to understand.

Yes, it can feel so scary to address this head-on, but dealing with the problem at the outset is way less painful than missing something or taking longer because you didn't understand fully. People are usually willing to help if you ask early, but they might be frustrated if instead you nod along and pretend.

Reframe your thinking from *I don't understand and I don't want anyone to notice* to *I deserve to understand*. That shift is key. Managing adult dyslexia isn't just about the strategies – it's about having the confidence to start using them.

Ways to better control the conversation in meetings

It's always easier to control conversations in one-to-one settings rather than large group meetings. But even in group settings, you can take steps to manage the flow of information.

Here are some options based on your confidence level:

Confident options:

- Be the person who creates the agenda and runs the meeting.
- Take notes and say, 'Sorry, before we move on, can I repeat what I've got so far?'

Medium-confidence options:

- Ask the person running the meeting to summarise each section – position it as helping everyone.
- Ask clarifying questions or for examples, to slow the pace and aid understanding.

Low-confidence options:

- Ask for information in advance so you can process it beforehand.
- Ask for a clear agenda to follow during the meeting.

Strategy two: get the big picture

A working memory strategy that I really enjoy teaching is using big-picture thinking to support working memory challenges. It helps you to unlock your strengths and deal with your challenges all at once.

This strategy works because it gives your brain a framework – a context to hook details on to. When you understand the overall purpose or direction of a conversation, your working memory can process individual points more clearly and free up space for new information.

When something is first explained, the individual details can feel harder to process as you fit that information together and understand the connections in your mind. Your brain is using working memory space to build an overview or big picture while also trying to hold on to all the individual details. If you can start with an overview or an explanation of what you are going to learn, it's much easier to understand and less taxing on your working memory.

So if someone starts talking and you're thinking, *What on earth is going on?* – you're probably searching for context. Here's what to say:

'Before you go any further, could you give a quick summary of what you want to talk about? I find that when I know the context, I'm able to understand the content better.'

Why getting an agenda or overview helps

A common dyslexic reasonable adjustment is receiving a meeting agenda in advance.

Here's why it matters: meetings often involve a flood of information. Having an overview of the topics or context can be essential to keeping up and understanding how everything interconnects. In large group meetings, where it's harder to control the conversation, the big picture becomes even more important.

Even a simple agenda can help you follow what's going on. The more detail it includes, the more valuable it becomes.

Tip: it's important to remember that not every meeting or every situation will require a full overview. Try to focus on the ones where you really want to show up confidently and won't have many chances to steer the conversation.

Strategy three: repeat and reformat

Here are two simple, powerful techniques to support your working memory: 1) repeat and 2) reformat.

Working memory is short-term – it's meant to pass information into other areas of the brain. Repeating something helps move it along. Reformatting it – into a visual, story or analogy (something dyslexic people love to think in) – makes it even stronger.

So when someone is explaining something to you and you feel overwhelmed, pause and ask them to repeat back what you have heard. This helps you process and open space for new information. (It can also help you remember names.)

When to use these strategies:

- When someone is giving you directions. Say: 'OK, so it's turn left, then second door on the right...' Don't worry if you get the directions wrong on the first repetition – just keep going until you get them right.
- When you need to remember something important and you aren't able to write it down.
- When you have to process a lot of information in a short time period to be able to give a clear answer. So for example, say: 'Before I give you an answer, can I just repeat everything to make sure I haven't missed anything important?'

Phrases I often use to reformat key information include:

- 'It sounds similar to...'
- 'So another way of thinking about it is...'
- 'So basically...'

Tip: if you're an especially visual thinker or love interconnections (as many dyslexics do), lean into that. So for example, if something reminds you of a TV show, find a way to introduce that concept to reformat the information. Don't shrink from being different: learn to own it, as it helps your brain hold less and communicate more. If you need an extra dollop of confidence to do this, chapter 16 explores the value of this style of thinking.

Strategy four: seek word recall support

Word recall can be deeply frustrating. It's often a sign that your working memory is getting overloaded, either due to feeling tired or too much going on around you.

When it strikes, use the waiter analogy: drop some information off and come back for it another time, if possible. However, if it happens at an important time and you need to manage the situation, the key is to move on and stay calm. That way, the word or concept will come back.

Instead, people tend to over-apologise, trying desperately to force the word out. This only heaps on the pressure and makes it even harder for your brain to retrieve the lost word.

I often tell clients to start trusting their brain more. I am all too aware of how ridiculous that advice sounds – doing so feels deeply alien for most dyslexic people. But pressure works against you.

Calm and confidence are the skills to learn – not speed.

When it happens, I like to move on as quickly as possible, using a line like: 'Oh, I lost my train of thought – you keep going and it will come back to me.' No pressure and no long silences. And the word always comes back.

Strategy five: use filler phrases

Managing working memory is about slowing down and giving your brain time to process without stress. This skill can be particularly important to master when it comes to processing questions or formulating an answer.

That's where filler phrases come in. They buy you time to understand the question before you start formulating your answer – preventing overload and confusion.

Examples of filler phrases:

- 'Oh, good question.'
- 'I haven't had that question before.'

- 'That definitely requires some thought.'
- 'Let me think that through.'
- 'I've got a few thoughts coming up on that.'

Buying yourself 10 seconds of breathing space can make all the difference.

Strategy six: word vomit and then recap

This strategy is for those moments when you feel like you've rambled – like the client who stopped speaking mid-sentence out of embarrassment.

Dyslexic people are often verbal processors. We require time to think through our thoughts aloud before we can clearly and simply break them down. However, there are times when you don't have time to prepare and need to share your thoughts raw.

The goal here is to focus on your recap. Don't worry about how the idea comes out at first. Let yourself ramble a little to unpack your thoughts, then wrap it up confidently after your working memory has had a chance to process.

Here is a step-by-step overview of this concept:

1. **Be honest that you're speaking off the top of your head**
   Saying something like: 'I think I have an idea, but it's just off the top of my head, so bear with me as I try to break it down.' Or: 'I have a few thoughts that are coming together. I want to break them down and then summarise.'

2. **Ramble for a bit**
   Think aloud and break down the thoughts that are coming into your mind. Focus on getting the idea out, not on perfection. Worrying about how you sound only drains your working memory capacity further.

3. **Recap strong**

   Signal that you are clear on your thoughts and you feel confident in your ideas. Use phrases like:

   - 'I had to break down my thoughts there, but basically...'
   - 'Thank you for letting me think that through. In summary...'
   - 'OK, so what I was trying to say was...'

Why this works

This strategy allows your working memory to break down an idea, process your thoughts fully and then recap with greater clarity. Often, it's only the ending that people actually remember – and when you give your brain a little time to verbally sort through your thoughts, that ending becomes clearer, more concise and more impactful.

What I often see people do instead

The ramble can feel uncomfortable, but what often happens is much worse: people stop halfway through breaking down their thoughts, worried they're not making sense, or avoid starting altogether due to past bad experiences. But it's only *after* the ramble that your brain has had a chance to process – and that's when you'll be most articulate. Stopping short robs you of that clarity.

Strategy seven: use tech to help you

Software is getting better and better at supporting dyslexics, and one of the biggest improvements has been in meeting recording software. These tools allow you to stay present and focus on what is happening, rather than splitting your working memory between listening and note-taking.

However, I do think it's important to stress that the goal of working memory strategies is to help you focus and engage *in the moment* –

not just understand after the event by watching the recording. If you're attending a one-hour meeting and then rewatching the full hour again, that's not a sustainable strategy.

For this reason, I believe successful working memory strategies need to allow us to understand and focus in the moment and where needed use recordings as a safety net for details.

Tip: choose tech that includes searchable transcripts or, even better, AI-generated summaries. This allows you to find what you need quickly and efficiently, without rewatching everything – making the recordings a safety net, not a second workload.

Strategy eight: use chunking

Chunking helps reduce the load on your working memory by grouping information with something familiar – something you already know and understand.

Here are a few examples of chunking in action:

1. **Remembering names**
   Link a name to someone you already know or a famous person – e.g. 'Natalie' reminds you of Natalie Portman.

2. **Remembering blocks of information**
   Use mnemonic devices – like the rainbow song – to group and recall larger sets of information.

3. **Instructions or directions**
   Instructions or directions are tough because they're unfamiliar. But if you anchor them to a known landmark ('Turn left at the shop with the red awning'), your brain has less to hold and more to connect.

How companies can support strategies for working memory issues

Working memory strategies don't just work for dyslexic employees – they improve meetings for *everyone*. Modern meetings are overloaded with detail, and most people struggle to keep up. Adjusting how meetings are run across the board makes them more inclusive, impactful and engaging.

1. Provide agendas and overviews

Clear agendas or goals for each meeting will help dyslexic employees process key information – and ensure that goals are met and key information is covered.

2. Follow up with key details

Allow people to focus on the overview during meetings by following up with specifics afterwards. This can be done via email, shared notes or summaries, depending on the situation.

3. Use company-wide recording software

Recording software for meetings is becoming standard. It is a useful tool to ensure key details aren't lost and people remain present. Having a recording process for *all* meetings will make the process less embarrassing for dyslexic staff and help everyone.

4. Repeat key points

When thinking about working memory strategies within meetings it's important to not just think about how people can engage with information after the meeting, but also helping people feel clear during the meeting. One of the best and most simple ways to do this is through repetition of key points or details. This helps key points be processed fully and not missed, should working memory be overloaded.

5. Include breaks in long meetings

Working memory fatigues easily and once its capacity is reduced, it can be really hard to process new information or remember instructions. Schedule in breaks where possible, particularly in long meetings.

6. Offer second screens

A second screen on desks or work stations can make a huge difference, because it means you are no longer having to hold information in your head and overly rely on working memory. Instead, it allows people to review instructions while completing a task. This can significantly reduce mistakes and the effort required to complete the tasks. Dyslexic adults consistently report this as a game-changer.

10
Interviewing

Chapter summary

Why this chapter is important

Interviewing is one of the common challenges dyslexic adults face. It's also a great way to demonstrate how multiple dyslexic challenges can co-occur. In interviews, we're managing working memory, confidence, processing speed, non-linear thinking, and many other things besides. These challenges rarely have a single solution – they need resolving through micro-strategies, layered together.

The strategies we are going to explore in this chapter don't just apply to job interviews – they're relevant in other high-pressure situations, such as:
- Speaking on panels.
- Explaining yourself at a doctor's appointment.
- Being a witness or speaking to police or in a court.
- Speaking to a journalist.

What you will learn

- How multiple dyslexic challenges can be a problem simultaneously.
- Strategies to communicate clearly in stressful situations.
- How to discuss dyslexia confidently and effectively in interviews.

Why is interviewing such a big dyslexic challenge?

In chapter 4, I referred to the backpack metaphor: dyslexic adults carry invisible bricks that slow us down and make life harder. Interviewing is a perfect example of how those bricks stack up. It's not just working memory and non-linear thinking – it's also the fear of judgement, not knowing what support you need, and pressure to perform.

Here's an overview of the specific challenges that can be associated with dyslexia and interviewing:

1. Lack of understanding of what you need

In interviews, you often sense something is wrong – you aren't speaking as smoothly as you'd like or you're forgetting key details, and deep down you know you're not performing at your best. But figuring out why that is happening and what strategies might help can feel really difficult – especially when there is limited information out there for dyslexic adults.

It's no wonder many of us avoid interviews altogether. We might decide not to change job or go for a senior position, afraid they may involve an interview that'll spotlight our weaker areas. Or when we're pushed into high-pressure situations like interviews, we may need to spend hours preparing to help calm nerves or stand half a chance of presenting ourselves well.

> **Real-world story**
>
> Before one of my biggest interviews, I was in exactly this position – doubting myself and not really believing I could fully express myself successfully in an interview. But I wanted to move to London, and that meant changing jobs, so I had no choice but to go for the interview.

> The interview fell on a Monday and because I was so nervous and unsure of what strategies might work, I felt like I had to spend all weekend revising and prepping. This meant I skipped a long-planned visit to a friend and instead spent hours watching YouTube videos on interview tips and writing and rewriting notes on what I might say, hoping I could memorise them sufficiently to feel confident.
>
> I see this all the time with clients who are in the process of interviewing – putting life on hold to learn and rehearse scripts, hoping that will be the fix. But in reality, it often leads to overload and doesn't build confidence.

2. Lack of confidence

Confidence is essential for managing dyslexia successfully. I know I have said this before but it's so important, it's worth repeating. Confidence helps reduce stress, lowers cortisol and strengthens working memory.

Having confidence also allows you to remember and actually *use* your strategies – slowing down conversations, asking for clarity and processing information better.

Without confidence, embarrassment kicks in. You can find yourself shrinking because you're afraid of not understanding something or stay quiet when you're confused.

3. Working memory and stress

Working memory is already a challenge in multiple areas of our lives but when stress is involved, it weakens further. This makes high-stress situations like interviews even harder. Here is how it can impact you most in interviews:

1. Processing two-part questions

Interviewers love nothing more than multiple-part questions, such as: 'Can you tell me about a time you were able to show your leadership skills, and what it taught you about management?'

Answering these questions can quickly overload your working memory and lead to a feeling of being a deer in the headlights. You might get halfway through answering and then forget the second half of the question.

2. Ordering and organising answers

Answering interview questions is increasingly becoming a science. Interview formats like STAR (Situation, Task, Action, Result) require you to remember the question (which is often in multiple parts), think of the story you want to tell and recall how to formulate the answer. That's a working memory nightmare – and can quickly overload your brain.

3. Remembering all the key details

It's not just the structure of the answer that your brain has to contend with, but all those pesky little details and statistics that help show the value. Your brain is having to hold on to multiple elements at once just to answer one question:

   I. How to answer part one of the question.
      - What example you want to share.
      - How to format the answer correctly.
      - Any details required to make the example sound impressive.
   II. How to answer part two of the question.

No wonder we so quickly get caught out!

It's at moments like these when you find yourself saying completely the wrong thing and so confused you can't even say when your birthday is.

> ### Real-world story
>
> While writing this book, I took on a new coaching client. She was intelligent and articulate and had recently completed her master's degree, so I assumed she felt confident managing her dyslexia and didn't let it hold her back.
>
> However, she told me she hadn't pursued a major career qualification because an interview was required as part of the process and she believed she 'couldn't' do it. This didn't shock me – I have heard it many times.
>
> I challenged her ideas and reminded her of the work she'd put into her master's and how hard that probably felt at first. We talked about building systems and strategies. Yes, it might be hard – but she was clearly capable and with the right strategies, everything would feel easier.

4. Non-linear thinking

Interviewing means thinking on your feet. Dyslexic people can be great at this, but the challenge is that we are complex thinkers. We see the big picture, make connections between different topics and think in stories or images – not always in neat sentences and words.

In interviews, breaking down complex ideas can feel overwhelming, especially when you're required to do it without any warning.

It can be easy to create a narrative that we are 'incapable', but in fact your brain is *too* capable. The ideas and concepts we come up with are just not suited to the speed and simple, clear structure required in interviews.

5. Not knowing how to talk about dyslexia

Dyslexia is often a source of frustration and stigma. Bringing it up in an interview – when you want to put your best foot forward – can feel really nerve-wracking.

I've been there: starting new jobs, feeling unsure if it's a good idea or not to disclose my dyslexia, scared of being judged. I felt so confused, frustrated and alone. That's why I created Dyslexia in Adults – to offer clarity, confidence and tried-and tested strategies. I wanted someone to confidently say, 'Do this', rather than me just guessing all the time. Now I'm the person providing the advice.

> ### Real-world story
>
> I once interviewed for a role that was a huge step up in my career. I was both nervous and excited about the opportunity. As part of the interview process, they asked me to review a task in a test environment in their office and then present my ideas to them.
>
> I hadn't told them at this stage that I was dyslexic – I was concerned that if I did they would judge me and think I was incapable. I also didn't really understand what strategies would help me; I couldn't pick apart how dyslexia would show up in this moment and what I needed to support me.
>
> Looking back, having extra time, not judging my work by my spelling mistakes and getting context in advance would probably have made a huge difference and helped calm my nerves. Instead, I fretted constantly over how little time I had, which made processing the test difficult. As a consequence, my presentation afterwards was a little clumsily ordered and confused in a lot of the phrasing. I even remember one of the senior directors pointing out a spelling mistake, which made me go bright red and feel embarrassed for the rest of the interview.
>
> Luckily, my idea really impressed them. They saw my potential – even if they didn't know the challenges were related to dyslexia. But I later found out I was significantly underpaid compared to others at a similar level. If I'd had a chance to build a plan, feel confident processing the information and not been embarrassed by my spelling, who knows how much better I could have done – and how much more I would have been paid.

Strategies when interviewing

Interview formats can vary depending on the context – from informal chats to multi-stage assessments with structured tests. They might take place at work, in a court of law, in front of a panel or in a studio. So, the strategies you need should flex with the situation. Think of them as a toolkit: use what you need, when you need it.

Strategy one: process the question

As dyslexics, there is often a gap between hearing something and truly processing and understanding it correctly. Yet processing a question as quickly and accurately as possible is essential when you're being interviewed. It allows you to give your best answer – avoiding you replaying the moment the next day and wishing you'd answered differently.

Use filler phrases

Much of managing dyslexia is about slowing down and doing things one at a time. So when you're asked a question, you need to process it first before you build a reply. But no one wants to sit in awkward silence for five seconds. This is where filler phrases are useful – they buy you time to process what you have heard and ease pressure.

Here are a few good examples:

- 'Yes, I thought about this question a little this morning.'
- 'I have a few good examples – let me think which fits best.'
- 'I haven't had that question before – let me think through what might work.'

Choose phrases that sound natural to you. The goal is to make them automatic – so they don't drain your processing power.

Repeat the question

Repeating the question can be another way to buy time to think through what you have heard. As we discussed on p. 141, repeating helps move information out of working memory and into long-term memory.

Here are some examples:

- 'Just to confirm, you're asking...'
- 'Let me repeat that back...'
- 'So, a time I showed leadership and what it taught me about management was...'

Again, the key here is to make it sound as natural to you as possible – a subconscious habit that allows your brain to focus on processing the question.

Request questions or topics in advance

Requesting interview questions or topics in advance is a common and reasonable adjustment in most situations. It's important to remember that a job interview is about allowing you to show what you're capable of, not a raw memory test. Knowing what questions you'll be answering or topics will be covered can allow for clearer thinking and stronger answers.

Asking for questions or topics in advance can feel uncomfortable but this is where confidence and changing your way of thinking about managing dyslexia comes into play. Reframe the request as a way to perform at your best.

> ### Questions in legal settings
>
> Of course, other types of interview might be different. For example, in legal settings, especially court proceedings, the goal is to gather spontaneous, truthful recollections. It is usually not possible to request questions in advance, in order to preserve the integrity of the answers and avoid any chance of coaching or bias. That said, you're legally entitled to ask for reasonable adjustments and support. For more on your rights in the UK, go to: https://www.gov.uk/government/organisations/hm-courts-and-tribunals-service/about/equality-and-diversity

> In other countries, a quick google should provide you with the information you need.
>
> In these situations I recommend you lean on the other approaches I have mentioned, such as repeating information, writing down key points and allowing yourself to think through your response on paper before responding.

How to ask for questions or topics in advance It doesn't have to be scary. Here's a simple, confident script you can use to approach it:

> 'I want to let you know I am dyslexic. To ensure I'm able to answer questions to the best of my ability, previous companies I've interviewed with have provided the questions or topics in advance. I'd be grateful if you could please do the same.'

I like this approach because it normalises the request by highlighting that past companies have been happy to do it. Even if it's not true for you personally, it's true for lots of other people – and you can borrow that confidence.

The law is on your side In the UK, many large companies already use standardised interview questions to reduce bias and comply with UK equality legislation. This makes it easier to ask for adjustments or flag concerns. If a company doesn't comply with these standards, they may be breaching The Equality Act 2010 – and frankly, failing the vibe check of being somewhere you would want to work.

Many other countries have similar equality legislation, including the USA, Canada, New Zealand, South Africa, Sweden and others. Do your research and learn what your rights are – knowledge is power, after all.

Write notes during the interview

As mentioned previously, slowing down is a core strategy during interviews. One simple, effective way to do this is to write down the question, then jot two or three points for your reply. This reduces working memory load and helps you feel confident in your response.

It's important we flip the switch around dyslexia: bringing a notebook and jotting down the question or your thoughts doesn't make you look incapable – it shows you're thoughtful, strategic and committed to giving a clear, considered answer.

Everyone in the room wants you to do well and answer the questions to the best of your ability. Any employer worth your time should welcome a few scribbled notes if they help you achieve a clear answer.

Of course, the challenge here is writing while thinking and reading while speaking. So I recommend you write only short joggers.

Let's use the example of the multi-part question from earlier:

Question: 'Can you tell me about a time you were able to show your leadership skills, and what it taught you about management?'

You might write:

Show leadership + learnt management

➡ Managing the launch project

➡ Lead project management meeting

➡ Problem with junior employee

This helps you process what you have heard, remember the question and stay on track if your mind blanks or gets overloaded. Make sure it's as digestible as possible.

Strategy two: form clear replies

When formulating replies off the top of your head, the challenge can be how to order and plan your thoughts succinctly. Interviews often require structured answers – like STAR or competency formats – which adds challenge as you try to mould your response into that structure.

Bring notes

Bringing notes to an interview can be a powerful way to reduce mental load. It allows you to think about the order and structure of your example beforehand. Having clear notes you can quickly refer to also means you don't need to worry about forgetting key facts and figures.

The same rules apply to prepared notes as to writing notes in the moment: keep it brief! Reading dense text is not a dyslexic strength, so aim for high-level joggers that give you the big picture of how you want to structure a story, or key facts and figures you want to include. You'll likely need only one or two words per key concept.

Here is what I recommend you prepare:

- A detailed note about your strongest examples, which you know you will mention.
- Important statistics or outcomes for other examples.
- A list of successes to pull from if your brain goes blank.
- Questions for the employer (so you don't have to hold them in your memory).

This gives you a safety net. If you lose your train of thought mid-story, you can pick it up easily or if you can't think of what to say, you have a list of your key stories in one place. You'd be surprised by how much bringing notes boosts your confidence – so much so, you may not even need them.

Important reframe

For many dyslexics, bringing notes feels like you're revealing you have 'a bad memory', but the reality is that well-prepared notes make you look organised, prepared and the kind of employee anyone would want. We shouldn't hide the effort we put into our work – it's something people genuinely value.

> ## Real-world story
>
> You may think keeping the information in your notes brief is a bit obvious, so here is an example of how overdoing interview prep can make forming your answers harder, not easier.
>
> One client came to me after failing three rounds of promotion interviews in the fire service. He said he was confused as to why he was struggling to remember everything, as he spent hours before each interview practising and repeating his lines.
>
> The word 'lines' caught my attention. His biggest concern was that he didn't articulate himself well, so he had written full paragraphs for every possible question and was hoping to remember it each time. We quickly ditched these and switched to short bullet-point notes instead.
>
> Whereas previously he'd felt bringing a notebook would show him up, this time he took it. This, coupled with asking for the questions in advance, meant he passed the interview. He is now a chief fire officer.

Understand if the job is right for you

A specific challenge for dyslexics is trying to assess if the job – and the organisation – you are interviewing for will actually work for you. There's often discomfort around being honest and uncertainty about how to assess the environment, but it's a vital part of the process.

Be honest about your dyslexia

These ideas have been woven throughout this chapter, but here's a reminder of why it's better to be open and honest about your dyslexia in the workplace, and in any other situation that involves an interview scenario.

Support helps you do your best

You're trying to be successful and represent yourself well. It's better to get support and feel capable than to say nothing and want the ground to swallow you up.

Tip: ask for a morning interview if possible – so your brain is fresher and processing is easier.

Find out if a company or organisation will value you

If someone judges you for asking for support or is rude about your dyslexia, it's better you find out now. You'll always be dyslexic even if you try to mask it, so it's worth knowing upfront what kind of company or organisation you're dealing with.

In the workplace, think of your abilities and the value you offer as specialist skills. A dyslexic person can do any job or role, but not every individual is right for every job or role. There's a subtle distinction – and it's OK that you aren't a perfect fit for every company. You just need to figure out which is the right one for you.

If you don't feel supported or comfortable in how the organisation is dealing with your request, this is a red flag and your signal to walk away. You deserve a workplace or environment that supports you.

Ask questions

Many clients have told me: 'I said I was dyslexic and they said it was fine and they would be supportive – but when dyslexic challenges came up, it wasn't fine.' Often, when people say they are fine with your dyslexia and will provide support, they don't really know what they are agreeing to.

So although I think it can be valuable to disclose your dyslexia if you feel the situation is right and you're confident enough, there are better ways to figure out if a role is right for you.

Here are some questions I recommend asking:

- 'What does success look like in this job?'
- 'What style of management do you use?'
- 'What's a past mistake someone in your team made, and how did you handle it?'
- 'What proofreading processes do you have?'
- 'How much autonomy will I have to approach tasks in my own way?'
- 'Have you tweaked any processes to support other individuals – and what are examples of that?'

Also ask about two or three accommodations you would find valuable and see what they say. Here's a script you can use:

As you know, I'm dyslexic. I've worked hard to figure out what support works for me, and I wanted to share a few of the strategies that have helped, to see if they'd be possible in this role:

- Proofreading important documents as standard.
- Planning and check-in meetings as part of my one-to-ones.
- A second meeting after project kick-off to aid processing.

This shows that you're capable and are managing your dyslexia well but also makes it clear that working successfully requires support at times.

How companies can support strategies for interviewing

Interviewing is one of the most common dyslexic challenges that people are aware of, so many organisations have already taken steps to improve accessibility. However, having to be the one to ask for support can still feel embarrassing. These small changes can make a big difference:

1. Standardise support

Instead of relying on the individual to advocate for their needs, companies should offer standard support for dyslexic and neurodiverse candidates.

This might look like a link to accessibility options in every interview invite. Companies could also offer a pack outlining five key support options, with space for candidates to request additional adjustments.

Solutions like these would make the process less stressful and remove the burden of self-advocacy.

2. Interviews don't need to be a memory test

Many interviews feel like exams at school, testing memory rather than getting to the bottom of someone's skills and discovering their value. But for many jobs or roles, it isn't a good memory that demonstrates skill in the role.

Where possible, provide questions and topics in advance. This allows individuals to think through their answers and give you their best.

3. Don't use two-part questions

Multi-part questions are a nightmare for dyslexic candidates. Instead, ask the questions separately and repeat longer questions. This is a simple and quick shift that can really help the person answer effectively.

11
Executive functions

Chapter summary

Why this chapter is important

If you're struggling with organisation or feel that you're constantly 'dropping the ball', then this is the chapter for you. 'Executive function' is a term that every neurodiverse person should know. They are the missing piece of the puzzle for many, especially when challenges feel confusing and don't seem directly linked to the reading and writing aspects of dyslexia.

What you will learn

- The root of many of the challenges that are associated with getting work done.
- Simple or quick strategies that help you move through your task list.
- What 'visual processes' actually mean when it comes to managing your to-do list.

Executive functions and the dyslexic brain

Think of your prefrontal cortex as your organisational assistant. It's there to help you navigate situations rationally and plan things well, to ensure they're done on time and thoughtfully.

I find dyslexic people often fall into two broad categories:

1. Organised but stressed.
2. Disorganised and embarrassed.

Neither is better or worse – but each involves quite different challenges.

Personally, I am 'disorganised and embarrassed'. For years, I struggled with executive functions without realising. I blamed myself and believed I wasn't 'good enough' and if I just 'tried harder' I could have got better.

Dyslexic people who are organised but stressed may find that although fewer mistakes slip through with planning and organisation, the time and effort they are having to spend can have a huge impact. This can lead to more burnout, less time in your life to do things you enjoy and a constant feeling of stress and anxiety.

Once I understood more about executive functions and their impact, everything became easier because it was no longer about shame – it was about strategies.

Here are the 11 primary executive functions:

1. Planning and prioritisation – figuring out what to do first.
2. Time management – understanding the passage of time.
3. Working memory – holding information in your head for short periods of time.
4. Organisation – organising concepts with ease and consistently keeping this up.

5. Impulse control – not saying something you shouldn't or not thinking through your thoughts before speaking.
6. Task initiation – getting started on tasks in a timely manner.
7. Metacognition – evaluating and reflecting on your situation or actions.
8. Emotional control – staying regulated and calm.
9. Flexible thinking – being adaptable or changing your thinking.
10. Sustained attention – focusing on only one task at a time.
11. Goal-directed persistence – sticking with long-term goals.

Issues with executive functions are commonly associated with ADHD, but they affect all neurodiversities – including dyslexia.

Common dyslexic challenges with executive functions

1. Procrastination

Task initiation is one of the biggest dyslexic challenges my clients tell me about. For many people, it can feel impossible to get started on something – tasks sit collecting dust at the bottom of to-do lists, or hours pass before you get going on a piece of work, which means you then have to work extra hours to make up for the time you spent avoiding it.

Difficulties with getting started often leave people stuck in the mantra of 'I just need to try harder', but this is a perfect example of how better systems would help you work smarter.

2. Breaking down tasks

This is one of the biggest dyslexic challenges and it's important to understand its impact. Because we are big-picture thinkers, it can be easy to lump information together and not be able to simply and easily break down all of the individual elements that come into a task. A simple task can quickly become overwhelming and feel impossible. Executive function issues are a primary culprit in this problem. Here are the two key difficulties:

I. **Organising thoughts:** Breaking down thoughts and organising them is such an important part of planning for dyslexics. However, this requires time and clarity, and may feel really difficult. Everything can quickly get into a mess and become overwhelming, meaning we skip this stage and jump straight in without a plan, making everything harder.

II. **Managing time:** Without a clear plan, managing time and understanding how long a task will take becomes extremely difficult. A one-hour task becomes three – and still isn't done. This leads to the feeling that you're always behind and never on top of your work.

Real-world story

I recently took on a mentorship role for dyslexic entrepreneurs with Virgin StartUp. During one session, I was speaking to one of my mentees, and she told me that while she was in training a coach had spoken about the importance of business planning. However, what she said to me was, 'I don't think I am going to do business planning – it feels too overwhelming.' I knew exactly what she meant, as I had fallen into the same trap with my company Dyslexia in Adults: there were too many areas to think about and organise my thoughts around, so it felt easier to just figure things out day to day. For both of us, it felt like too much to think about and too many unclear thoughts to organise so it was easier to ignore the problem.

What I've learned over the years, though, is that although messy action can work for a time, eventually not making a plan can keep you going in circles. To help my mentee avoid this, we talked about how to make business planning feel more accessible to her and how to get started in a way that didn't require breaking down too many complex ideas. Once we had simplified the approach she was able to get started and make a plan rather than just using avoidance as a strategy.

3. Managing workload

Managing workload when you're dyslexic can feel like a constant battle. Keeping track of what you need to do and finding an approach to make it happen often feels like a full-time job due to executive dysfunction. Here's how it often shows up:

- **Task overload** – planning and prioritising feels like doing mental acrobatics.
- **Difficulty sticking to plans** – distractions from instant messages, emails and meetings can derail focus, especially for tasks where there is no clear deadline.
- **Last-minute panic** – deadlines are essential for managing executive functions better; without them, working towards a long-term goal can be difficult and you can feel like you're constantly just firefighting the work right in front of you.
- **Post-it-note city** – scattered scraps of paper with different ideas jotted on them and to-do lists stored across different notebooks make it hard to consolidate tasks or build a visual system.

Strategies for executive functions

There's no silver bullet for managing executive functions, but a collection of small, strategic shifts can transform how you manage your work. Each of these strategies interlocks with another: managing workload helps with task initiation, and starting tasks on time makes managing workload easier.

Strategy one: stop procrastinating and get started quicker

Procrastination can eat up your day more than you like to admit. But it's not laziness – it's your brain working against you. It doesn't want to get started, it doesn't want to understand a task and it doesn't like sitting down to plan. Expecting yourself to be better next week won't work without a strategy.

I say that firmly because for many of us, struggling with these challenges and the criticism that comes alongside them means we internalise shame. And even though you may know it's not true that you're 'not trying hard enough', you still believe 'trying harder' is the solution. But actually, it's having better systems that will change your reality. Here are four that can really help:

1. Accountability

The neurotypical view of task initiation is that our brains should be able to figure out what is important or what needs to be done and get started straight away. However, the challenge that comes with neurodiversity is sometimes that importance alone isn't enough of a motivator for us to get going; we need to add other tools to build up the ability to start a task. One useful option can be accountability.

An example of this is when your house is a mess and it's only when you know your friend is coming over that you finally do the dishes. We all know we 'should' do things, but sometimes it's only the external accountability of your friend seeing your pile of dishes that finally sparks the interest.

The same can be true for the task sitting at the bottom of your to-do list that you are currently ignoring. Having outside motivation can be hugely helpful to spur you to get going.

Body doubling is a valuable neurodiverse tool for accountability that can easily be achieved without anyone knowing. It just means having someone alongside you while you get things done, to hold you accountable.

Here are some ideas for how you can do it:

- Call a friend while you tidy the kitchen.
- Tell your boss, partner or a friend what you're doing today.
- Co-work with friends and colleagues via video conferencing.

Use accountability when you have something you know you 'should' do but don't feel like doing. I use it when a deadline feels remote or realistically I know my brain could quickly come up with a reason not to do a task.

If you hear yourself say *I should . . .* or *I want to . . .*, it's time to make a plan, to make the plan happen.

For example, I was nervous when writing this book that I would do all the work near the deadline, as that is my usual mode of working when it comes to managing big projects. Instead, I set up weekly check-ins with my team to make sure I was moving forwards.

2. Big win v little win

Getting started can feel daunting, especially when a task is clumped up into one huge task. There are two schools of thought when it comes to getting started. I will lay them both out, along with their benefits. You can then try both and see which one works best for you:

- **Little win:** Start with a few small tasks to build motivation and help you feel ready to tackle bigger chunks. Personally, I start each day writing my to-do list, then I write a few easy emails and then dive into big projects when I have built up motivation.
- **Big win:** A lot of people call this 'eat the frog', which means tackling the biggest task first. This reduces the mental overwhelm that big tasks can cause, meaning you can get going straight away.

3. Pomodoro method

Sometimes staying focused on a task can feel almost impossible; all your brain wants to do is something – anything – else, especially if the task is boring or cognitively challenging. The pomodoro method is a great way to continue working through a project that feels hard while giving your brain structure and breathing space.

Here is how it works:

- 25 minutes of focused work
- 5-minute break (use an alarm)
- Repeat for 2 hours
- Take a 15-minute break
- Repeat

4. Fake deadlines

This is my favourite strategy, which I use with my neurodiverse team: everything must have a deadline.

> **Deadlines are key motivation tools; without them, nothing gets done. Things languish on our to-do list and drain mental energy.**

My advice is to set a pre-deadline with someone other than the people you're delivering the work to (i.e. send an important presentation to your mum/friend two days early for proofreading). This shifts the urgency forwards and makes the deadline feel more real.

I wouldn't get anything done without this strategy. It's been a total game-changer for me.

The reframe here is instead of believing that you 'will try harder next week', you build the deadlines your brain needs to achieve tasks.

Strategy two: break down tasks and plan ahead

Having a firm grasp of your tasks – either at work or in your personal life – is vital. It helps you manage time, avoid forgetting things and get started faster.

As dyslexics we always feel frustrated that work takes us longer than expected, which can lead you to thinking you need to 'get started straight away' and don't have time to waste on planning. But instead of thinking planning is going to eat into your time, you need to flip the switch and see it as saving future you time.

Here are a few strategies to help you:

- **10 minutes' planning saves an hour** – break down the task into its parts before starting.
- **Request help** – dyslexics are often external processors, which means it can be harder to do planning and prioritisation alone. Ask others to help you get started and point out where you have underestimated the time required or missed an important task. Say, 'Do you mind if I talk through my plan?'
- **Brain dump** – another option for verbal processing is brain dumping everything in no particular order. That could be a voice note, to Large Language Models (LLMs) (such as ChatGPT), on a whiteboard or in a notebook. By just writing a list of everything that is in your head you will be able to process it quicker, plan and prioritise next steps and feel clearer about the work required. It doesn't have to be well ordered – it's just about getting everything down and then building a plan.

Strategy three: keep track of your tasks

Managing your workload better is not just about knowing how much time something is going to take – it's about having a full picture of what you have to do and when. Many dyslexics track tasks in a scattergun fashion, but consolidation is key.

Here are a couple of ideas to help with that:

1. Use visual systems

How many times have you heard that dyslexics need to have visual systems? But often with advice that has been said a hundred times before, we understand the concept but don't really know what it means and how to use it in real life.

Let's change that. Here is what 'visual systems' really means:

I. Seeing everything you need to do in one place.
II. Seeing urgency and time frames for each task.
III. Seeing the break-down of each task once you start.

It's about freeing up your brain from having to *remember* everything, so you have the capacity to *think through* what needs to be done.

If you're trying to remember the time of your haircut and what time you need to pick up your child from school while also planning how many hours you need to write a report, it's easy to understand how your brain can get overwhelmed.

Whereas if you can see in your calendar the time you have available in between your haircut and school pick-up, you can quickly plan how to use those three hours to write the report.

Tip: a Kanban board (a project management tool) is a great way to lay this out. Most productivity tools use this format – and it's what I rely on daily.

2. Use to-do lists

To-do lists are lifesavers for so many reasons. They help you:

- Break down tasks.
- Offload working memory.
- Stay on track when your brain feels scattered.

No wonder they're often recommended to support executive functions challenges. Let's talk about how to best use them:

I. **Brain dump everything on to your list** – get all your thoughts out and make sure you have everything in one place. Clear your working memory of everything.
II. **Prioritise** – identify what needs to be done today and what can be done later. Ideally, there should be no more than three priorities, otherwise you might struggle to make a plan.

III. **Visual overview** – sketch out your day: what the plans are and how you're going to organise them.

Tip: use two lists – one for daily tasks and a longer list for longer-term tasks.

By committing to one central location for all your thoughts and tasks, you'll start to rely on it instinctively. It soon becomes second nature and helps you create consistency in your strategies rather than feeling like you're starting a new plan every few months.

Consistency is always difficult, but the more regularly you can do it, the better. I recommend that you 'habit stack' this task: write your list while you drink your morning coffee or on your daily commute.

> ## Real-world story
>
> I can't stress how much organisation is my arch nemesis. I'm a lot better than I used to be, but it's not easy for me. Here is how I manage my to-do list as a busy founder:
>
> - I use a Kanban board in Notion.
> - I keep it updated to the best of my ability, reminding my team that if it isn't on my task tracker, 'it doesn't exist'.
> - Even then I find myself accidentally keeping track of things in my head and inevitably forgetting, and every time I do, I say, 'I should have put it on Notion.'

On top of that, whenever I get busy I brain dump to make sure I haven't forgotten anything and I have a clear vision of what is going on and what is due. The busier I am, the more I rely on visual planning and breaking my day and week down into task blocks.

Sometimes people who don't know me well think I'm organised. Those who do would never say that! But that's the power of a system.

Strategy four: manage your time better

Figuring out *what* you have to do is half the battle. The other half is knowing how *long* something is going to take you. Many dyslexic people underestimate time – and then fall behind.

Here are some simple strategies for how to build better time awareness:

1. Plan backwards

Planning backwards is an obvious, simple strategy that you may have tried before and forgotten about, so here is a quick refresher, illustrated with a story:

A client came to me because he was struggling with time management. We talked about planning backwards and its value and he admitted he doesn't really do it. So we started with what he was doing that evening: going to his aunt's house after work.

Here's how it went:

Goal: arrive at aunt's house at 7 p.m.

Breakdown:

- Walk to the aunt's house: 10 minutes (probably 5 minutes, but rounding up never hurt anyone).
- Go to the changing rooms and faff about getting ready: 10 minutes.
- Work out: 1 hour.
- Walk to the gym: 10 minutes.
- Transition from work to the gym: 15 minutes (transitions are often very difficult for neurodiverse people, so don't underestimate this one).
- Finish work: 5.30 p.m.

He thought 1 hour 30 minutes was enough. It wasn't. Seeing it all laid out and being honest about the time lost in transition helped him push his arrival time at his aunt's back to a more realistic 7.30 p.m.

Tip: planning backwards can feel unnecessary, but it can save you lots of stress and reveal pockets where you're losing track of time.

2. Monotask

When you struggle with time management, multitasking can make this challenge even harder. So let's think of multitasking as a myth.

Instead, try to figure out how to implement monotasking: doing one task and then starting the next one.

What you need to do:

- **Keep a to-do list beside you** – jot down ideas there instead of trying to do 20 small tasks alongside your project.
- **Know your headspace** – do you require deep focus or are you in admin mode? They are different types of activity and need to be done at different times.
- **Acknowledge your focus levels** – if your focus wanes, get up and go for a short walk rather than starting a new task.
- **Use stimuli** – some dyslexic people also have ADHD and may need stimuli to stay focused. That doesn't mean doing 20 tasks at once – it means listening to engaging music or changing your environment.
- **Block your days by task type** – this keeps the focus on what you should be doing that week and how you should think about your week. For example, ensuring I don't book calls at the start and end of the week means I don't eat away at my focus. Here is how I organise my week:
    - Monday: important projects.
    - Tuesday: coaching calls.
    - Wednesday: running the business/team one-to-ones.
    - Thursday and Friday: project work.

3. Track and analyse where you're losing time

Time can sometimes feel either like it's going at a million miles an hour or each second can feel like a lifetime, with nothing in between.

Figuring out what is going on and where you're losing time is so important. The following are helpful:

- Use timers to see what you're spending your time on.
- Map out rough timelines and then test them.
- Try to do something the same way a few times before changing your approach, so you can spot what is going wrong.
- Take some time to analyse your day and see what took longer than expected. This will help you figure out your next steps and where you need to build in contingency. Sometimes unexpected things crop up – your train is cancelled, your child has to be collected from school, your parent needs your help – and if you don't build in any flex at all, you can easily fall behind when life clashes with your schedule.

4. Use alarms

Time management often boils down to *now* or *not now*, which is where alarms can help you keep track of time. Here are a few examples of situations where an alarm might be helpful:

- You need to leave the house in five minutes. That is *not now*, so you feel like you have a lifetime ahead of you to go on side quests. *Tip: set an alarm for the time you need to start preparing your bag and finding your keys so you leave on time.*

- A doctor's appointment is later this afternoon. Although this is *not now*, it feels like it will be happening soon, meaning you can't get on with your day for fear of forgetting. This is called 'waiting mode'. *Tip: set an alarm for when you need to get going so you can focus on other things and don't spend all day worrying and in waiting mode.*

- You have a meeting in 10 minutes. This is *not now*, but because it's only 10 minutes away, you're in waiting mode and can't get

started on another task. Instead, you wander to the kitchen and get distracted by a cleaning side quest that takes 15 minutes and you end up being late to the meeting.
Tip: set alarms for 5 minutes before and 1 minute before the meeting.

5. Say no

Let's be honest, for many dyslexic people, saying no feels hard. We want to show people we're capable – and we're so used to working harder than most, a little extra feels like an easy yes.

But piling on more without a clear sense of what you're doing, and when, is a recipe for failure. Instead, we need to get comfortable with saying no. Doing so isn't a 'failure', it's about protecting your headspace to allow you to do everything to the best of your ability.

Saying no can take a lot of confidence but it also requires processing speed. When you're presented with information, you need time to figure out what work it entails and how much time the task will take. It can sometimes feel easier to just say yes rather than asking for that time to think it through and then give your answer.

To help you do this, here are some scripts:

- 'That sounds like a great idea. I would like to take it away, map out the task and come back to you with feasibility and timelines.'
- 'There are a lot of competing priorities at the moment. Let me get a full scope of the task and see if I have capacity.'
- 'I've found in the past that blanket yeses can be unhelpful for managing priorities. Can I give you an answer tomorrow?'

These scripts buy you that time to truly process what's being asked and assess your workload realistically.

The important reframe here is switching your thoughts from *I have to say yes otherwise they will think I can't do my job* to *By managing my priorities carefully I am able to do my best, which is what everyone wants of me.*

How companies can support strategies for executive functions

Executive functions challenges are a perfect example of what this book is about: redefining what is 'easy' and changing how we can see people who struggle with certain tasks as being incapable or not valuable. Simple shifts in attitudes and systems can make a huge difference. Let's take a look at some now:

1. View task management support as reasonable

Many neurodiverse people struggle with breaking down tasks and getting started, which can have huge ramifications if they're not supported correctly. Reasonable accommodations include simple steps like attaching deadlines to all tasks or supporting with prioritisation in one-to-ones.

> **Real-world story**
>
> A senior manager in a high-powered job that I once spoke to was close to being put on a performance review – not because they weren't capable, but because they weren't managing their workload.
>
> Instead of offering support and structures, their boss had said to them, 'You're too senior to need this kind of help.'
>
> This mindset is exactly what we need to challenge and change.

2. Use company-wide organisation software

There are countless organisational systems that can help with the visual planning that is required for dyslexics and neurodiverse people to better plan, organise and prioritise their work. But many companies restrict access to these tools and offer no alternatives in their own systems.

Either companies need to create policies for allowing individuals to work with IT to add tools quickly, or offer a broader range of planning software company-wide.

3. Allow time for questions

Over and over again I see managers expecting their team to be given a project and then deliver with no opportunities in between to clarify anything or ask for support. Management is often bolted on to someone's role – and they don't have time to support or manage people properly.

Building in time for questions or clarification can really reduce procrastination and help with time management.

12
Slow processing

> **Chapter summary**
>
> **Why this chapter is important**
>
> It's easy to build the narrative that you are 'slow' – either slow at doing tasks or slow at picking up new information. That sense of everything taking longer, knowing it's due to dyslexia but not understanding *why*, can be really frustrating. You feel like you don't have control over your brain or a plan that actually works.
>
> In this chapter, I break down why you may take longer to explain yourself or find it difficult to fully understand a topic straight away – and offer useful strategies to manage this more effectively.
>
> **What you will learn**
>
> - How to feel less exhausted by processing information.
> - How to learn new information efficiently for your brain.
> - How to manage having a million ideas that feel difficult to explain.

Understanding slow processing

You're focused. You've heard every word someone has said. But you leave the meeting or conversation thinking, *I don't really understand what's going on*. That's slow processing in action. It's common in dyslexic people and it can feel frustrating, embarrassing and like you're 'stupid' because you can't get to grips with something in the time frame allocated to it, or only come up with responses after the event. But here's the truth: your brain just needs more time.

In this section, we'll break down all the ways slow processing can impact you so you have a full understanding of when, and what, strategies might help.

1. The fear around slow processing

For many dyslexic people, receiving new information can feel like a rabbit-in-the-headlights moment. You're focusing more on trying to *look* like you understand than actually *processing* what's being said. Perhaps you try your best to focus on the small nuggets that you can understand and maybe write down – but working memory means you can't write and listen at the same time.

So you just 'get through' the interaction without clarifying anything, for fear of revealing your slow processing. Afterwards, you're confused about what to do and feel unsure what questions to ask to help you move forwards.

> ### Real-world story
>
> I mentioned my client in the previous chapter and how she struggled with processing a new project and breaking down her thoughts.
>
> She worked in consulting and was constantly given new projects and tasks to quickly get up to speed with. Information

would fly at her and she couldn't process everything in the first meeting. Her questions and clarity came *after* the meeting, when she'd done a bit of work. She came to me with her confidence crushed and worried consulting wasn't for her. She couldn't clarify everything to do with the project and ask important questions simultaneously.

What she realised she needed was a second 'check-in,' either remotely or in person, depending on how many follow-up questions or clarifications she needed. The biggest game-changer was proactively asking for this upfront. Instead of feeling she had to just end the meeting and hope for the best, she said, 'Everything initially makes sense. I find I have more questions when I get back into a task, so can I message you/book in a call for next week?'

Think about processing like loading little soldiers into your brain one by one, not in groups. A whole army can fit – it just takes time.

2. Not coming across how you'd like

People often want ideas or thoughts straight away, which can be really difficult when you are dyslexic. Slow processing speed means we often need to take something away, to really digest everything and build up our big picture before having our best ideas.

So when you are first speaking to someone about a new project you might feel like you aren't able to speak as clearly as you would like or have clear thoughts and ideas, since you are still building out your understanding.

For example, someone asks you for an update but you only remember half of what is needed or it's only once you get going that you start to remember additional facts or elements. You need time to 'get into' a task before your thoughts fully surface.

3. Procrastinating

When we don't understand something fully or are frustrated by the process of breaking a task down, procrastination kicks in. This is covered in more detail in chapter 11.

4. Saying yes without thinking it through

You agree to tasks before you've had time to process what the new work entails and what it means for your existing workload. It feels easier to say yes and figure the rest out later.

5. Exhaustion from processing

It's not just about *how long* something takes – it's *how much it costs us* and how we feel after we have worked hard at a task. For many dyslexics, processing something verbally or in writing can be draining, making other tasks that may need to be done that day feel impossible. This leads to fear and avoidance of these tasks because they seem so difficult to achieve.

6. Good ideas come the next day

Slow processing can mean that ideas, thoughts or questions come to us only after a conversation has ended. It can feel embarrassing to follow up with an idea or question at a later date.

Understanding non-linear thinking

Slow processing often makes you feel 'stupid'. You're not. And you can reframe your dyslexia by understanding the role *non-linear thinking* plays.

> **Dyslexic people are complex thinkers. Instead of thinking in neat straight lines or isolated compartments, we see the big**

picture and all the interconnections between the elements. Building up that rich picture takes time and effort – and *that's* an important part of why processing is slower.

So, non-linear thinking can be a huge strength. But there are a few problems associated with it:

1. You stray off-topic

Everyone's discussing an idea or problem but your brain has jumped to a different topic entirely – because you can see a connection. This is what helps us come up with solutions or ideas that feel original and unique but it can also make engaging with topics more complicated.

Some people can also feel like you're being rude if you appear to ignore the topic under discussion and jump to something else, if they don't understand that you're just exploring alternative angles. This can rub people up the wrong way, so it's important to understand this and why it might colour their reaction to your response. You can mitigate it by prefacing your words with 'I'm just looking at this from a different angle: how about . . .' For more on this, *see* 'Build a bridge to your ideas' on p. 190.

> ### Real-world story
>
> One of my clients was a classic dyslexic ideas person. In meetings, her brain flooded with solutions and ideas, but they didn't always neatly fit the meeting's structure or agenda. So she would stay quiet and submit her ideas after the meeting had finished. But it was too late – decisions had often been taken before she'd had a chance to contribute, or she felt that people weren't always able to see her value or ideas.

2. You struggle to order or break down your new ideas

Your brain constantly generates new ideas. But they come so easily and quickly and are so complex that they often don't have a simple start or end point and can be hard to break down. This means it can be difficult to communicate them effectively.

Strategies for slow processing

Slow processing and non-linear thinking are close bedfellows – they often impact each other. Here are some strategies to help you manage this challenge and build confidence in how your brain works:

Strategy one: fully understand concepts

We often talk about 'learning' as something that happens in school but that's far too narrow and simplistic. Processing and understanding new ideas happens every day, whether it's the latest family drama your mum is telling you about over dinner or a new task from your boss.

Feeling like you fully understand something – quickly or clearly – is a core skill for dyslexic people to master. Here are different strategies to deploy in different situations:

1. Break down your thoughts

Flipping the script and seeing your brain as complex is essential for managing processing speeds differently. Your brain wants to build that complexity to understand something fully – which means breaking down your thoughts before you construct a plan.

Here's how:

- **Write everything down** – anything connected to the topic and anything circling in your brain. Don't worry about the order; just keep writing until everything is out.

- **Order or group thoughts** – this is where mind maps make sense. Dyslexic people love to group topics once we've broken down ideas. This is when you can start to spot gaps or problems.
- **Plan and prioritise** – once you have a full visual overview of everything, it's easier to prioritise and plan next steps.

What are mind maps?

Mind maps are visual representations of information and ideas. You start by writing or drawing the main idea in the centre and then draw lines to branch out to related topics, details and subtopics – a bit like a web. You can then use colour coding to pick out themes or words. They are very useful for organising information and showing how ideas connect to a central concept.

2. Ask for the big picture

Dyslexic strengths can sometimes feel like weaknesses, especially when building the big picture takes time. Here are some suggestions on how to 'speed up' the creation of the big picture and make you feel capable and confident:

Request an overview Standard dyslexic advice – which I also gave earlier – is to ask for an agenda before you go into a meeting. That's helpful, but a better way of thinking about it is that you are trying to build an *overview* – of the meeting, project or even a story someone is about to tell you.

Whatever the situation is, that overview will help you process the individual details more easily and quickly.

Find out the why Understanding *why* or getting context behind a decision or process helps build that complexity and big picture we need. Getting more information is key, even if it feels overwhelming.

Try these phrases:

- 'Can you give me an example of that?'
- 'Can you give me the context behind that decision?'
- 'What was the thinking that led to this situation?'

Ask the questions that make you feel stupid

Sometimes we have nagging questions that stop us fully understanding a topic, but the years of negative comments and lack of trust in our brains can make us afraid to ask. I have also heard people say they worry about 'being annoying' for asking questions that don't feel socially acceptable.

The reframe here is that those questions are valuable. They will help you understand better and create insights, for *everyone*.

Strategy two: explaining your thought process

1. Explain things the way your brain sees them

Dyslexic people think in images, stories or analogies. That's often how our ideas come to us. Yet we often try to translate them into the 'neurotypical way' – making life harder for ourselves.

Sharing ideas exactly how you see them will be much easier and help you communicate better. Narrative reasoning is a dyslexic strength. Talking in stories, as we touch on in section three, is a technique that helps people connect to our ideas.

2. Build a bridge to your ideas

Although ideas are a classic dyslexic strength, most people struggle to see their own ideas as *unique*. They assume others see the same connections or that the idea is so obvious they don't need to explain it.

But people don't see what we see. Having unique ideas means you need to explain your perspective. You need to take people on the journey you have gone on in your mind.

I like to call it 'building a bridge'. When you start telling a story or idea, first explain how you got there. Set the scene with the image you have in your mind and then dive into the brilliant new thing you're ready to drop.

Strategy three: managing your energy

Strategies are not just about being able to do a task faster. The real test is: *do you feel capable*? Are you no longer avoiding tasks because you trust yourself to do them? That's the goal and the bar I set for myself and for my clients.

Managing the *energy cost* of a task is key. If you find processing information or learning something so difficult you can't form a sentence well for the rest of the day, it's no wonder you feel negatively about yourself and what you are capable of.

So here are some examples of how to process new information without feeling like you've just had a lobotomy.

1. Verbal processing

Dyslexics find a lot of value in repeating back or verbally processing what they understand. This can create the connections and big picture we so desperately crave and helps something really make sense. It is often a much less mentally taxing way of getting to grips with something. Here are some ways you can do this:

Teach someone I firmly believe that teaching is the best way to truly understand a topic. It forces you to think in a completely different way and can help build up the connections or simplify a topic, which is something we value as dyslexics to help process something fully.

Of course, there are classic options like training a new starter or running a lunch-and-learn session, but it doesn't always have to be this structured – maybe you try explaining something to your partner to see where your gaps are. It might feel daunting, but it really works.

Use voice noting Send yourself voice notes. Dictate your thoughts. There's something about the accountability of knowing you're doing a voice note that makes you actually break down an idea – even if it's messy or doesn't fully make sense yet. It can foreground themes and clarify what you don't fully understand.

Have whiteboard sessions Processing your thoughts visually on a whiteboard before starting a new project or idea is invaluable for dyslexic people. Make this a standard part of your routine. It will help you reduce procrastination and feel less exhausted.

Call a friend Sometimes I call a friend and say, 'I hope you don't mind, but I need a couple of minutes to talk through my thoughts – then I think I'll come to an answer myself.' You don't necessarily need their input – you just need the space to break down your ideas.

2. Take more regular breaks

Not all tasks drain you equally. Processing-heavy tasks will take more from you, more quickly. Be honest with yourself about this and make sure you're taking the breaks that you need to keep going or to feel capable.

Having to flex your systems and break patterns is part of managing dyslexia. It's important to do what is needed to manage this particular task – not what you needed last time. And try not to beat yourself up for needing more.

How companies can support processing strategies

Throughout this chapter, I've shared the realities of processing information in a dyslexic-friendly way, separating each part of the process and presenting information in bitesize chunks.

For some organisations, this break-down might be frustrating or difficult. The extent to which this might need to be done will vary by individual and situation. This is an example of exactly why we need to recategorise what 'easy' looks like and be OK with differences in how people respond.

1. Simple changes go a long way

Starting with an overview and then allowing time for questions after the initial meeting are small adjustments that can make a big difference. These steps help dyslexic employees access their brains' full potential – and give you the value you're looking for.

2. Think about how you deliver important information

Remember: some 700 million people worldwide are dyslexic. We're not talking about helping just one or two people – we're talking about supporting a large portion of the population.

And in today's fast-paced world, most people struggle to process large volumes of written information. So taking the time to ensure things are explained well and carefully will help a significant number of people – not just dyslexics.

3. Build a culture of productivity

When companies focus on *productivity* rather than hours worked, it becomes easier for employees to take breaks and allow themselves to reset – which is vital for dyslexic professionals. Taking breaks allows information to settle in, and the net result is that employees will be more productive.

13

Reading and writing

> **Chapter summary**
>
> **Why this chapter is important**
>
> As much as I've tried, it's very hard to fully avoid reading and writing in any job or everyday life. That's why, instead of dodging our challenges, we need to build robust and valuable strategies that reduce the mental load and allow our strengths to show. That is the goal of this chapter: to help you feel confident and capable when it comes to the classic dyslexic hurdles.
>
> **What you will learn**
>
> - How to read and process information as efficiently as possible.
> - How to order and organise your thoughts in writing.
> - How to check your work in a dyslexia-friendly way that minimises mistakes.

Understanding challenges with reading and writing

We all know that dyslexia makes words feel unnatural to us. That feeling when you open a long email or someone asks you to read aloud and your gut goes *NO*.

But it's not just the task – it's the shame that can be rooted in this challenge due to the endless red lines through homework or being laughed at for mistakes in the past. This history can make getting started or even engaging in this work feel unnatural.

Reading challenges

Wherever you go and whatever you do, at some point, you'll need to read. Whether it's a sign on a door, instructions for making up baby formula or taking medicine, an application for your child's school, navigating a train station, or dealing with a work email – reading is a required skill.

But just because it's everywhere doesn't mean it's natural. In fact, the act of encoding language is deeply *unnatural*. Entire degrees are built around the gap between the *signifier* (the word) and the *signified* (the thing or concept it represents). Reading isn't just decoding letters – it's translating symbols into meaning, and that's a cognitively demanding task.

1. Processing the text

I can read every word. I can process each one individually. Actually understanding what the text *means* feels beyond me sometimes.

It's frustrating when you can't tie the individual words together to form the story you know they tell. You can read it over and over again and yet it feels like nothing has gone in. You misread instructions, misunderstand expectations and feel stuck before you even start because it just doesn't make sense.

Saying the words aloud can be helpful, because it makes engaging easier, but you need to balance this with the increased energy cost. It can definitely be helpful for shorter pieces of text, though, so it's worth trying if you are on your own and the situation and time allows it.

2. Embarrassment about reading speed

It isn't just about comprehension – just following each line feels like wading through treacle. This means I read slower, which is hard enough, but then my brain goes into hyperdrive and starts asking: *How long is normal? How long am I allowed to take?* If someone hands me their phone to read a message, I feel like I have to calculate the 'acceptable' time to read it before handing it back.

So I scan. I skim over a document and don't read it fully or, if I do really try to engage in understanding the text, I only get through half of it – and pretend I've read more than I really have.

> ### Real-world story
>
> At a big tech company, meetings would often start with silent document reading. This felt totally alien to me. No one had explained the big picture, what was important, which section to read first and what all the acronyms meant.
>
> I spent more time worrying about how I could *pretend* I had read the document than really engaging with the content. It felt easier not to try than to start and have to stop partway through – and then have to deal with the embarrassment I would feel.

3. Reading out loud in front of others

Is there anything worse than having to read out loud in front of others? You skip words, misread phrases or add in words that don't exist. The longer it continues, the more stressed you get, and the worse it gets.

> **Real-world story**
>
> A client told me that he was asked to read aloud in a meeting. He wasn't prepared and got a bit shaky, causing someone in his team to laugh. This triggered memories of school and how embarrassing it was, and he ended up needing to make an excuse and go to the bathroom to compose himself. He told me that since that moment he has avoided speaking in meetings altogether.

4. Not reading books

Reading books requires a lot of mental effort. I'm lucky if I read one book a year and even then it feels like a constant struggle. It's only really possible when I'm on holiday and have the mental energy.

I'm acutely aware of all the knowledge I must have missed out on and the stories I haven't heard. Thank goodness for podcasts and audiobooks – they've opened up a world of information that was previously locked away from me.

5. Misreading small details

Managing dyslexia often feels like you can't trust your brain – that eventually you'll make a mistake. There are countless examples of dyslexic people misreading dates, confusing train times and struggling with airport signage – it's exhausting to feel constantly let down by your own processing.

Writing challenges

Writing, like reading, shows up everywhere in life. Even if your job doesn't involve much writing, modern life still demands it – from endlessly filling in forms online to registering at the dentist, managing your banking, buying a house or writing a will.

And then there's the everyday writing: WhatsApp groups, social messages, work emails, project updates, further education assignments, career qualifications – the list goes on.

Thankfully, technology is starting to make life slightly easier for dyslexic people, but many pitfalls remain. And more often than not, we approach writing tasks with a legacy of shame and fear weighing us down and undermining our confidence.

Here are a few common examples of writing challenges:

1. Writing a long document or piece of text

Ordering your thoughts, structuring your sentences and checking spelling – it's a triple threat for dyslexic people. Getting complex thoughts down in a clear order can seem impossible, especially when you try to do it all at once because you feel like you're behind. Most people try to cram everything in at once, rushing to catch up. But that approach often leads to overwhelm, confusion and burnout.

2. Small mistakes that people understand

How many times have you received a reply to a message or an email with an asterisk correcting your grammar? They understood what you meant – but still felt that your mistake was unacceptable and wanted you to know that.

What I find so perverse about these situations is: if you understood and it doesn't matter, what's the problem? Especially when the impact of these little corrections can be huge embarrassment for the person you send them to. It isn't necessary or kind.

> ### Real-world story
>
> One coaching client told me she felt she wasn't good enough for her role, even though she was a senior director at one of the biggest companies in the world. Sadly, this is a common feeling among dyslexic professionals who struggle with what they think are 'basic' tasks. For this particular client, it was her challenge with writing reports that was undermining her confidence.
>
> They would often take her a couple of hours, which made her feel frustrated. She couldn't see the effort it took to collate the project updates, break down complex ideas, craft persuasive phrasing and showcase the value of her work. She just berated herself for the time they took and wished it could be easier or quicker. She felt that 'successful' people or non-dyslexic people should be able to write these reports quickly.
>
> Her goal, like most people with these issues, was to do the reports 'quickly' and she would tell me that she was too slow. These are comments I have come to realise are built around shame we have had from an early age. So I asked her to quantify what time period she would like to create such complex documents, and she answered around an hour and a half at least. As soon as she said that her next words were, 'I guess I am not really that far off at all.' It's amazing how shame can cloud the reality of how capable you already were.

3. Grammar and phrasing in bigger documents

Grammar and phrasing can be a challenge for dyslexic people, too. We might switch tenses and use inconsistent terms, or write in a way that's confusing. We also often over-explain or fail to break things down clearly. It's not laziness – it's the cognitive load of translating complex thoughts into linear language.

Overall approach for reading and writing strategies

Before implementing systems, we need to understand the theory behind what works and what doesn't. Here are two foundational problems that block people from progressing:

1. Low confidence and shame

People's perception of their reading and writing challenges and the reality are often vastly different. Many have built up a picture of themselves as slow and prone to making mistakes, thanks to past shame and frustration.

A big part of making progress is separating the shame from the actual problem, so we can figure out what is reasonable and what is something we need to let go of.

Whatever you're working on, start by setting clear goals:

- What do you want to achieve?
- What is a 'best case'?
- How long should processing a document take?
- How many books will you read a year?
- Which emails *must* be mistake-free – and which ones can slip through?

Without these boundaries, shame will make the entire process harder.

2. Things move too fast and there's too much information

Dyslexic brains struggle with doing too many things at once. That's why much of managing dyslexia is about splitting apart tasks and doing one thing at a time.

Here are a few reminders I use myself:

- If you're reading an important document, turn off notifications and use noise-cancelling headphones.
- If you're writing a text to someone, finish it before answering the question your kid/partner has shouted at you. Otherwise, it will make no sense.
- It's OK to pause in silence for a few seconds to write something down. I used to feel awkward about this – but it's essential.
- When reading dense documents, separate the overview from the micro-details. Do one read for the overview, then another for the specifics.

Strategies for reading and writing

The overall approach for reading and writing strategies is to reduce overwhelm. In the following strategies we look at how to pull apart each element of the process to allow your brain time to think.

Strategy one: write the overview first, then the sentences

Writing, like reading, works best when tasks are separated. Start by building the outline of what you want to say first and then worry about the individual sentences later.

Separating ideas from words is essential. Take time to think through your concepts before diving into sentence construction. Our brains are complex – mapping out what we want to say first allows the sentences to flow.

Personally, I just dump all my jumbled thoughts into LLMs and let it do the writing for me. That way, my brain focuses on what it does best – generating ideas – and lets AI handle the structure and polish.

How to create an outline

- **Verbal processing** – use a voice note or talk to a friend to get all your thoughts out.

- **Brain dump** – write everything out in any old order.
- **Group and order** – once everything is out, start grouping themes and building structure.

Tip: for more complex ideas, verbal processing first can be helpful.

Strategy two: how to process text when reading

This section is about how to really feel like you have understood what you've read.

Build context

I know I must sound like a broken record at this point, but dyslexic people love the big picture and building an overview in our minds of what we are reading. So instead of letting information develop step by step, do a first read of a document or ask for an overview of what you're going to read. This makes it easier to place the individual details within the overview.

Tip: where possible (and allowed), I love to use AI to get an overview of a big document before engaging with the details.

Reformat

Reformatting is one of my favourite ways to process something. It involves taking all the information in and then writing it out in a new style or connecting it to an image or story you already know. This helps it 'click' faster in your brain.

Reduce effort

These tips are about making reading less exhausting:

Seek quiet Background noise can make digesting text almost impossible. Personally, noise-cancelling headphones or going to a quiet place to focus really does make a huge difference. This is a great reasonable adjustment to request – especially as offices become busier.

Follow along with your mouse or finger It sounds trivial, but following along with your mouse and highlighting a sentence or using your finger is useful. It helps your brain stay away from its natural location of the big picture and really focus and engage with the detail that can feel so boring to engage with (hello, ADHD).

Choose the right time of day

Managing your day and energy levels is key. This is where accepting you have to do things differently comes into play. So if you need to turn around documents quickly, make sure you have time to do it in the morning, when your brain is fresh. I structure my day to make sure that important, cognitively demanding tasks come first.

Many neurodiverse people use something called the 'spoon theory' to help them prioritise and understand energy management when it comes to ordering tasks. By realising you only have a certain number of 'spoons' (units of energy) available to you in a day, you can decide what you 'spend' them on and how quickly you use them up. Basically, it's about assigning energy to the most important tasks first, and being realistic about the energy you have available.

Use text-to-speech

Listening to a document while following along visually supports the multisensory learning that enables dyslexic brains to process quickly and efficiently. It is always really helpful when that text can also be highlighted at the same time as you are reading and hearing it, to further aid processing and focus.

What does radical acceptance look like with reading?

We don't have to be good at everything when it comes to dyslexia. It's OK to have areas that are weaker and need more support. So here is what radical acceptance may look like:

1. **Telling people you need longer to read** – this reduces stress and makes the task easier.

2. **Not needing to read everything** – it's OK to ask for something to be explained in a different format to make it easier to process.
3. **Accepting the effort** – acknowledging that reading requires energy and time helps you look at the problem differently and focus on the interventions, rather than wasting energy hiding the problem.

Strategy three: speak out your thoughts to help your writing

A common way of supporting dyslexia is dictation – but it isn't always straightforward. Many of my clients say the same: it helps, but there is a knack to using it correctly. Here are my tips:

- **Use it for spelling specific words**
  Don't rewrite an entire sentence just because you can't spell a tricky word. Dictating the word lets you access the intelligence you know you have, rather than limiting yourself to words you know how to spell.
- **Use it for low-effort writing**
  Writing isn't just about accuracy – you need to think about the energy it requires. I sometimes dictate messages to friends when I'm feeling exhausted (especially to ones who refuse voice notes!) or when I'm using LLMs and don't need the order to be perfect.
- **Ordering thoughts**
  When you're dictating long documents, it's important to start with a rough outline, otherwise you might quickly get confused and think this method doesn't work for you. It likely will, if you have a rough plan to help reduce working memory load.

Strategy four: create safety nets

Catching dyslexic mistakes in writing is hard. The small grammar or spelling errors that slip through – only to be noticed after you've hit send – are all too familiar.

My approach to this is: safety nets.

I want you to picture a trapeze artist doing incredible feats in the air. They don't want to fall but they know they have to plan for failure and have safety nets in place.

Your writing needs to be thought about in the same way. Work on the assumption that you will fall and plan how to catch those falls effectively.

In practice, how do we go about creating a safety net for our brains? Let's take a look:

Step one: recognise this as a hard task

As I said earlier, words aren't always our friend – they're not the thing we connect best with. This means that spotting small errors in a sea of text can feel very hard. This is key: we want these tasks to be easy, but the truth is that they're not easy for our brains. Expecting ease only adds to the shame and makes the situation harder than it needs to be.

Reframe – who decided this was 'easy'? (*See* p. 124 for a reminder about this.)

Step two: use checklists

Start by writing down the standard mistakes you make or the key elements you specifically want to look over. These might be mistakes that have been highlighted in the past or areas you know you particularly struggle with.

Tip: keep the list short – no more than five items or only important concepts – otherwise it will start to become unmanageable. Find the sweet spot between thoroughness and efficiency.

Step three: separate out things to check

Ideally, each item on your checklist should be checked *individually*. Asking your brain to juggle multiple things at once – especially when the task is already difficult – is asking for mistakes to happen.

Tip: if you can't check things one by one, the next best thing is to group certain tasks into *headspace type*. For example, don't check phrasing and grammar while also scanning for factual accuracy. Keep cognitive tasks aligned.

Step four: create headspace

When and *how* you check is as important as *what* you check. Getting it right will allow you to focus and engage with what you're doing. This may involve planning your checking process in advance to make sure you have time to do it well.

Here are some examples of how to support your headspace:

- **Fresh eyes** – check in the morning or after a break.
- **Quiet space** – use headphones or find a distraction-free place.
- **Change of scenery** – move to a new area to re-engage your brain.
- **Print it out** – physical copies can help you spot errors.
- **Remove distractions** – mute or turn off your instant messages, emails and notifications.

Step five: ask friends or family

Many dyslexic people have an incredibly supportive network of people behind the scenes who check documents and important text to spot things we might miss, especially when it comes to text that isn't specifically work-related.

Step six: use the right tech

Tech is revolutionising how dyslexic people manage difficult tasks – especially checking work. There are a few options here:

- **Grammarly** – this goes beyond spellcheck to help with phrasing, tone and those flabby sentences we write that can often sound confusing.
- **Text-to-speech** – by hearing something instead of reading it, we have a much higher chance of catching mistakes and realising what is wrong – especially with small errors like transposing letters ('angel' and 'angle').

- **AI** – unlike some overhyped assistive technology, AI has genuinely helped level up my dyslexia and made me feel confident about expressing my ideas more clearly.

Step seven: get support at work

For important documents, final checks should be done by *someone other than you*. That isn't just best practice for dyslexia, it's best practice for people in general. If a company or organisation doesn't have review processes and mistakes slip through, that's a *process error*.

But whether you're trying to change the process or get more support than is normally given (even if it would be good practice to do that anyway), remember to ask in advance for support with final checks.

Here's a simple script that will help you get the support you need:

> 'I often find that during the final stage of a project I spend a lot longer than I would like checking the document for small errors. I will of course do a thorough check but could we build in a final check process that means I'm able to work more efficiently?'

Planning ahead means you're creating a helpful process and being aware of your challenges, rather than spending hours working hard only for mistakes to still slip through. Doing it at the beginning makes it easier to manage expectations and schedule appropriately.

Creating your own personal safety net is a journey, not a destination. It takes time to build and iterate what will work for you based on your circumstances and what challenges you have with dyslexia.

But every time you start a task or a mistake arises, shift the narrative from *I am useless* to *Where did my system fail?*, and from *I need to try harder* to *What safety net did I not have?*

Focusing on the system, not the self, is essential for creating change and building better strategies.

Strategy five: how to deal with the grammar police

Don't you just wish that people would be kinder about small spelling mistakes, especially when they know what we mean? Sadly, many people still take good spelling and grammar as a sign of intelligence and hard work. Which is ridiculous when you think about what spelling actually shows about intelligence.

Here are some ways to handle the situation based on how you might want to respond:

1. Ignore them

Managing dyslexia is about building confidence in who you are and the reality of how your brain works and not centring your self-worth on how others treat you. If someone comments on spelling mistakes when they understood what you meant and it was an unimportant message then it's perfectly fine to ignore them.

This removes the shame you may feel and reminds you how much effort something took. That's what's important. It doesn't matter what they think and how they perceive spelling mistakes.

Best used for – WhatsApp messages or quick messages that people understood.

Important reframe – your brain finds spelling difficult, so if someone passes comment on a spelling mistake then it says more about them than you.

2. Tell them where to shove it

Sometimes there is nothing more satisfying than telling someone what you think of their comments about your dyslexia. Constant rude or unnecessary remarks can really land, and giving them a piece of your mind can be freeing.

Best used for – people who are trying to be intentionally hurtful and needlessly pedantic.

Important reframe – you're doing a service for the next dyslexic person they come across.

3. Explain your process

My personal favourite: kill them with kindness. This can be a really useful strategy, especially if you can't tell them where to shove it but you would really like to.

Here is how it works: instead of concealing your dyslexia, take a moment to explain the reality of your experience and the steps you have taken to get to this point. If I made a spelling mistake in an email, here's how I might phrase it:

> Hi Karen,
>
> I wanted to discuss the spelling mistake you pointed out in my email. I think it's important to explain that I am dyslexic and therefore some tasks that others would consider easy require extra effort for me. I do thoroughly check my work and use software to try to minimise errors, but due to the volume of emails I send and the time it takes to order and process my thoughts, small mistakes do sometimes happen. I try not to shame myself for this, especially when they don't materially impact understanding of the document.
>
> I will of course review my process and systems going forward, but I would be grateful if instead of pointing out individual errors we could instead focus on systems and strategies.

I believe that most people are ignorant rather than purposefully cruel. When they understand the steps you have taken and the reality of having a process and system, many will back down and cut you some slack.

Best used for – colleagues who may not understand dyslexia.

Important reframe – be proud of the systems and effort you put in to manage this challenge and remember that most people are not unkind – they're just unaware.

Putting the strategies into practice

It's impossible to cover every scenario where writing can be a challenge, so here are two common ones. The strategies apply to many other situations, too, so take the advice and see where else you can implement it.

1. Booking a flight or tickets

I think every dyslexic person is familiar with the panic of having to book something major – flights, expensive tickets or anything with high stakes and embarrassment if something goes wrong (remember my story about Lisbon on p. 21?).

Here's how to apply your safety net in this situation:

1. Accept this is a hard task and not something you should minimise. If needed, ask someone to sit with you or help you with it.
2. Write a checklist and check each item individually before clicking 'buy':
   - Airport codes
   - Flight dates
   - Flight times
   - Price
   - Number of passengers
   - Does the price include baggage?
3. Make sure distractions are removed and that you're focusing on what is going on.
4. When I booked my last flight, I screenshotted the details and dropped them into an LLM to ask if I'd missed anything before I clicked 'buy'. It might seem like overkill but it made me feel calmer and more confident.

2. Writing an email to the team

You've got a team-wide email to send that includes your senior managers. Your brain is doing anything and everything to put it off –

so much so that you did 10 other tasks that had been sitting on your to-do list just to avoid it.

Here's how to break it down:

1. Set a deadline for someone in the team to check your email by sending them a message: 'Would you mind checking my email for clarity and small errors if I send it to you by 4 p.m. tomorrow?' This builds accountability, provides motivation and creates a checking process.

2. Start with an outline and overview. Our brains struggle with complexity – separating ideas from sentence structure makes everything quicker and easier.
Tip: do a brain dump or verbal process to get down all of your ideas first. Ten minutes of planning can save you hours.

3. Once the outline is written you can focus on polishing the individual sentences and making sure grammar and spelling is correct.

4. Stand up, go for a quick walk, move to a quiet space, use headphones to reduce distractions. Then check:
   - Phrasing
   - Key accuracy issues
   - Spelling and grammar

5. Send it over to your checker. If anything slips through, you can explain all the steps you took and how diligent you had been.

How companies can support strategies for reading

I opened this chapter with the feeling you get as a dyslexic when you receive a long email, a document that is pages and pages long, or when someone sends you an article to read. An automatic *no* feeling that comes across your body – a gut-level resistance, knowing how much effort that task might cost you. The reality is that many people who are *not* dyslexic have the same reaction. Making changes to accommodate dyslexic employees will, once again, benefit everyone.

1. Consider alternative formats for presenting information

Often I think we default to writing because it feels like the option that we're most familiar with. But it's worth taking a second to think through how to present information and the options that are available. These include:

- Audio recordings.
- Short-form videos.
- Infographics and visual frameworks.
- Bullet-point summaries.
- Live walkthroughs or peer explanations.

> ### Screen-recording apps
>
> Screen-recording apps are something that many of my dyslexic clients really value. These apps allow you to record your screen with either a video or voice recording, helping you explain your point in a much more dyslexic-friendly way. Using a screen recorder makes it much easier to explain concepts simply without large amounts of text.
>
> Forward-thinking companies are increasingly using these kinds of videos for company updates or onboarding information, recognising that today's fast-paced world doesn't leave much time – or cognitive space – for reading long documents.

2. Allow space

Focusing on reading when it's the very thing your brain doesn't want to do is incredibly difficult. Having the right headspace to do it well is really important. For many, that means going to read in meeting rooms – often unavailable – or using headphones, which some companies don't allow.

Being able to focus without fuss or embarrassment on a task you already find difficult is invaluable. Companies need to make this easier, not harder.

3. Make reading easier

Of course not everything can be done without text, and there is always a time and place for written documents. When that's the case, here are a couple of simple ways to make reading more manageable:

- **Allow time** – intense time pressure makes reading harder. If something needs to be read quickly, try to send it in advance to give people time to process it.
- **Give the overview** – providing an overview of each section helps people build up the big picture first, which can be a game-changer.

4. Install software quickly

Reading and writing challenges are among the most recognised aspects of dyslexia – and thankfully, they're also the ones with the most advanced assistive tech solutions.

Yet often I hear from people who are stuck in long delays, waiting for employers to approve or install basic tools. In some cases, backlogs stretch over a year just to get simple tech signed off by IT. That's not just inefficient – it's actively harmful.

How companies can support strategies for writing

Writing can feel like an uphill battle when you're dyslexic – made worse when we are trying to fit in or hide how long it takes. This doesn't help productivity.

Although sometimes managing dyslexia can feel like it might be a hassle, the productivity gained through reduced procrastination and fewer hours spent hunting for small mistakes outweigh any perceived delay.

Here is how companies can handle this process better and support employees:

1. Create a checking policy

A team-wide process to check important documents will revolutionise the lives of dyslexic employees, removing shame, buying back hours of time and making achievable what can sometimes feel impossible.

2. Allow AI to be used

Adopting AI brings large-scale benefits for everyone, but the impact for dyslexic people will be particularly great. Blocking access to AI makes tasks more difficult across the board. It's like tying someone's hand behind their back and expecting them to perform at full capacity. Let them use the tools to access their potential.

3. Look at someone's overall value

Yes, some tasks do take dyslexics longer. But reviewing this in isolation – without considering the person's overall contribution – only adds shame.

We all know people have unique strengths and weaknesses, yet many workplaces still expect everyone to process at the same speed and in the same style. This doesn't reflect reality. It just reinforces stigma that doesn't help change anything for the better.

4. Look at systems, not 'hard work'

All too often, the managerial response to dyslexic challenges is: 'Just make sure you double-check your work.' This approach needs to end.

Instead, focus on building a system that works for the individual. Dyslexic people are often some of the hardest workers you'll meet. If they could have resolved the problem with hard work alone, they would have done it already.

Section Three

Unlocking dyslexic strengths

Welcome to section 3. Here, we'll explore how to understand and begin to unlock your dyslexic strengths.

The focus is on helping you see your dyslexic strengths in everyday life. Many of us can easily cite examples of the *challenges* dyslexia brings – but the same should be true for your dyslexic *strengths*. This section is designed to help you build up a clearer picture of how your dyslexic strengths are an essential part of who you are, and something to be appreciated.

I've intentionally chosen not to call dyslexia a 'superpower', as that framing is not relatable for many people. This isn't to deny the real value and opportunity that dyslexia strengths offer – it's about finding phrasing that feels authentic and closer to what you can relate to.

How to use this section

For many dyslexics I speak to, it can be hard to feel clear and confident about their strengths. Terms like 'big-picture thinking' can be hard to define, hard to explain to others and hard to recognise in yourself. In this section, we'll unpick why this is the case – and how to start reclaiming them. To do this, we'll break down the notion of dyslexic strengths into four areas, each with their own chapter:

- The truth about dyslexic strengths – and why we need to dismantle the 'superpower' narrative. Only then can we work on how to discover what your true strengths actually are and how you can showcase them.

- The strength of seeing the big picture – what this actually means and how it can be harnessed in our professional and personal lives.

- Other dyslexic strengths beyond big-picture thinking. Topics include image-centric thinking and 3D thinking, and how these can be useful.

- The final chapter is all about seeing the value of the dyslexic experience and how it shows up in real life. This includes acknowledging and celebrating the merits of the dyslexic strengths of hard work, resilience and emotional awareness.

14

The truth about dyslexic strengths

Chapter summary

Why this chapter is important

Many dyslexic people carry a longer list of struggles than strengths. This imbalance can make it hard to accept the notion that dyslexia brings value and opportunity. In this chapter, we'll first break down why dyslexic challenges may have blocked you from truly unlocking your dyslexic strengths. When we go into the detail of dyslexic strengths, those negative voices that used to block you will be silenced.

This matters because most dyslexics spend a lot of their time and energy focusing on managing challenges and not unlocking strengths.

But to truly unlock dyslexia, you need to spend time valuing and focusing on your strengths.

This can be hard to do when you feel like they don't exist for you or that you aren't clear on what to do with them.

> **What you will learn**
> - Why the superpower narrative is unhelpful and masks your true strengths.
> - How to prevent challenges clouding your strengths.
> - How to recognise and harness your own dyslexic strengths.
> - How companies can support dyslexic strengths.

The dyslexic 'superpower'

If dyslexia right now feels like more challenge than strength, or like your strengths aren't as bright and shiny as you want them to be, then you need to take a moment to dismantle the narrative of dyslexia being a 'superpower'. We touched on this earlier, but it's worth repeating.

Expecting dyslexia to be extraordinary might be the very thing stopping you from seeing its true value. The truth is: dyslexic strengths are often messy, sometimes subtle and occasionally mundane. They don't always magically appear the second you leave education. And they don't need to be extraordinary to be real. I'm not saying dyslexic strengths aren't exciting and valuable – I'm saying we need more realistic expectations of how they show up in everyday life.

Why the superpower narrative is problematic

There are many reasons why the superpower narrative is often part of the problem. Here are just a few:

1. The bar is too high

Calling dyslexia a superpower sets an unrealistic standard. It makes us search for examples that are grand and beyond normal expectations – overlooking and ignoring the everyday moments where dyslexic strengths actually show up, without fanfare.

When I work with clients, I ask questions about their work or personal life to uncover examples of these strengths. I commonly find that people ignore real successes that can obviously be attributed to dyslexia because they don't feel 'worthy' of the label of superpower. This is made even harder when they're too busy focusing on their challenges to see what their strengths have achieved.

> ### Real-world story
>
> One client, who was looking to change careers away from teaching to better match her strengths, spoke to me at length about being 'the dyslexic one' in a bookish, academic family. She was OK with being different but frustrated that she couldn't see the strengths that supposedly came from dyslexia.
>
> When we unpacked her dyslexic strengths, we identified countless examples of 'good ideas' she'd had by spotting opportunities and finding alternative ways to do things – but they just didn't feel 'enough' to warrant the label of being strengths. They felt flimsy when compared to the weight of the dyslexic challenges she experienced. She'd been waiting for a big, flashy win that made her feel worthy of having 'a superpower', ignoring the small, consistent examples of strength that had been there. After working together she decided to stay in teaching and now she regularly sees how her strengths are invaluable in her role.

2. It doesn't allow space for challenges

Dyslexia comes with challenges – real challenges that don't go away (especially when you don't have strategies that work). This can leave you feeling like you don't have any strengths because you're too busy dealing with the challenges.

But dyslexic strengths aren't inhibited by dyslexic challenges – it's better to see them as *coexisting*.

You might spend ages reading a document, then go for a walk around the block to digest it and suddenly have a genius idea with significant value. That doesn't mean the reading challenge wasn't real – it means the strength emerged alongside it.

One of the biggest challenges of acknowledging your dyslexic strengths is understanding that sometimes accessing the strengths themselves comes with huge challenges. For example, you might:

- Have a great idea but struggle to express it.
- See a solution to a problem but not be able to get started.
- Want to build the big picture but feel overwhelmed by the reading required.
- Have the ability to simplify everything – but not when it's all held in your head.

The key is to be able to recognise where your strengths end and your challenges begin. Otherwise, it can feel like you didn't get the 'superpower gene' that everyone else is raving about.

Real-world story

I had a client whose primary goal was to centre her career around her strengths. She knew she had great ideas but felt like they weren't having the impact she wanted. She told me about one idea she'd had about improving the processes for her team, which her boss had told her to speak to the director about. But she was holding herself back, worrying:

- *What if there's a reason I haven't thought of that makes this idea silly?*
- *What if my email has mistakes in it?*
- *How do I explain my idea in an email?*

> In the end, she sent the email and her director loved it. She messaged me a few months later to let me know her ideas had helped her get a promotion.
>
> In this instance, there was a positive outcome. But again and again I hear from people choosing to stay quiet and holding back their ideas because of fears about their challenges, such as communicating their thoughts or being unsure if they have missed something obvious. This is why to truly unlock dyslexic success, you need all three of the tools we have discussed: clarity in your strengths, confidence to say them and strategies to communicate them clearly.

If dyslexia isn't your superpower, what is it?

If you firmly disagree with me and think dyslexia should be your superpower – you like such a positive term and it feels connected with you and makes you focus on your strengths – then it has done its job and that is wonderful news. But if, like me, you want your dyslexia to have strength and value but the term 'superpower' just feels a bit cringe or overly simplistic, then this section is for you.

Rather than getting stuck on the phrasing, think of 'superpower' as a marketing tool for your brain. It's a term that's gained traction in the neurodiversity space and the positive message about strengths is starting to connect with the public and help turn the conversation around. Even if the term may have alienated you in the past, it's now a big global billboard for our brains and their value. You don't have to connect with the term itself, but you can acknowledge how exciting it is for the narrative to be shifting around neurodiversity.

That said, my suggestion is that you start to see being dyslexic as a 'difference that is neutral'; dyslexia is something that makes us different but isn't good or bad. The reason I choose the word 'neutral' is because sometimes the difference that dyslexia brings is frustrating and exhausting; sometimes it brings great opportunities and value.

I believe that when we step away from simplistic language such as 'useless' or 'superpower' to describe our dyslexia, we can have more honest and helpful internal conversations about being dyslexic. We can see the reality and nuance that comes with living with dyslexia without critical or overly positive language influencing this.

Dyslexic challenges don't invalidate dyslexic strengths

A big part of learning to unlock your dyslexic strengths is accepting that dyslexic challenges exist and trying not to see your dyslexic strengths as being invalidated by those challenges.

This section helps you navigate the messy reality of having both strengths and challenges, and how to stay positive and excited about being dyslexic even when things feel hard. Because when we let our challenges define our dyslexia, it robs our strengths of the space to grow.

So if right now you feel like you can't see your dyslexic strengths because you're so busy focusing on your challenges, here's how to pull yourself back to a more neutral, balanced perspective.

Seeing the full picture

When a dyslexic challenge sneaks in, it can be easy to catastrophise and feel absolutely awful about yet another embarrassing mistake. But it's really important to see yourself beyond that micro-moment and that mistake. Yes, you may have made a small mistake but you may have added huge value as well.

It can be so easy to fixate on a challenge and dismiss or reduce the value of any ideas or successes. Instead, try to separate them and see yourself not just as a mistake but as someone who brings value even if that did also involve a challenge. Step back and see the full reality of the picture. Ask yourself:

- Where have your ideas led to major successes that make a small spelling mistake insignificant?
- Where has your problem-solving prevented a catastrophe, making a missed deadline less important?
- Where has simplifying a complex document or task saved time – even if you procrastinated for a few days?

For example, you may have sent a meeting invite for the wrong date – an embarrassing and public mistake – but once you were at the meeting, you had an amazing idea that added real value. That amazing idea isn't nullified by the small clerical error.

Or else you may have been late to a friend's house because you got confused on timings, but when you got there you gave an incredible piece of advice that made being late totally irrelevant.

It all goes back to low-value and high-value tasks, again (see p. 76). What's the really important thing here – the small mistake or the great idea or piece of advice?

Dyslexic strengths need focus

When we talk about dyslexic strengths, we are looking for something that comes naturally to you or that you find easier than others. But a lot of the time, these strengths haven't had any focus or attention paid to them. Often this is because we feel like our strengths aren't what we need or aren't useful enough. This will only be made worse when, for many of us, we have rarely put much thought or time into learning how to hone these strengths, particularly when compared to the effort we put into dealing with our challenges.

Think of Michael Phelps: his physical traits – being double-jointed and having large hands – help make him a great swimmer. But that doesn't mean he doesn't have to train hard.

It's the same with dyslexic strengths. If you think about how much time you've spent learning to manage your challenges, just imagine what could be possible if you put the same effort into your strengths and properly focused on using the strategies I've set out in this book.

Here are a few examples of what going to the gym to work on your dyslexic strengths might look like:

- Learning how to best build up the big picture so you can access unique thinking faster and more consistently.
- Growing the confidence to speak up about your ideas rather than assuming someone must have already thought of it.
- Ensuring you select a job role or activity that is suited to your brain.

Coin theory: where there's a challenge, there's a strength

It's easy to compare ourselves to others – wishing we were more organised, more detail-oriented, faster at doing our work. Whatever it is, it can be easy to get stuck in comparison mode.

However, what I have come to realise is that a lot of the challenges we are so desperate to remove are often tied to our strengths. They're two sides of the same coin.

The most obvious example of this is how many dyslexics will be picked up on needing to be more 'detail-oriented' – they struggle with small errors. But the flip side is seeing the overview, being able to access the big picture – the patterns, connections and future possibilities.

This helps us reframe our challenges not as deficits, but just as indicators or what makes us different. It's not that we 'lack' something, it's that we have the other side of the coin.

Here are a few other examples of this concept in action:

- Difficulty processing may stem from being a complex thinker who likes to connect ideas and needs time to put these ideas together.
- Struggling with following a linear order means being able to reorganise structures and spot future problems.
- Confused sentences may push us towards visual and other styles of communication, which make connecting and persuading easier.

Coin theory helps us realise it's not that we have a deficit – it's that we have a different approach to these situations. Again, this reinforces the idea that dyslexia is a difference and that difference is neutral.

Challenges are easier to define than strengths

Dyslexic challenges can often feel more obvious and easier to identify than dyslexic strengths. That doesn't mean they happen more often, just that they're more visible. When you misspell a word, it's obvious it's dyslexia, whereas when you come up with an idea, it's harder to trace it back to dyslexia or even recognise it as a strength.

This creates a mental scorecard of thousands of examples of challenges, and only a few wins. But as you begin to understand, recognise and focus on your strengths, that mental scorecard can begin to even out – or maybe even tip in your favour.

Discovering your own dyslexic strengths

So far, we've explored how to shed some of the negative thoughts that can creep in when it comes to accepting and focusing on the value of dyslexia. Now I want to help you feel clear about how your dyslexia shows up in your life and career.

To make this easier, I've broken the process down into four simple stages.

1. Think about what you enjoy

It may sound obvious, but what we enjoy is often what we find easy – and what comes easily is very likely a natural strength or skill.

I often ask clients: 'What do you enjoy in your day? If you imagined yourself sitting having your morning coffee and saying, "I've got a great day ahead," what would that look like?'

The things that light us up are often the starting point for discovering our strengths.

Here are a few examples from my own ideal day and how they map to my strengths:

   I. Gossiping with friends about the latest drama ➡ great at problem-solving.
   II. Presenting at a conference ➡ simplifying complex ideas.
   III. Creating a new programme or offer ➡ spotting patterns and designing solutions.

2. Listen to compliments

When I finally figured out my dyslexic strengths, I started to realise that people had been pointing them out to me for years – but I had been so busy feeling frustrated, I hadn't had the capacity to hear them. That's why it's so important to listen to the compliments people pay you.

Chances are, the people around you have already noticed your strengths. Here are some common compliments and the strengths they reflect:

I. Big-picture thinking/connecting the dots

- 'I didn't think of it like that.'
- 'You always see things differently.'
- 'You always have good ideas.'
- 'I wish I could have your way of thinking.'
- 'I always find your advice so insightful.'

II. Simplification/visual thinking/narrative reasoning

- 'When you explain things, it always makes sense.'
- 'You have such a good perspective.'
- 'I always like your style of talking through concepts.'
- 'You're so good at persuading people.'
- 'Your presentations are so engaging.'

It can feel scary but asking people what they see as coming naturally to you can be a really good way of recognising and acknowledging your strengths.

Here's a script that might help you:

> 'I've been learning more about my dyslexia recently and I want to get a better understanding of my dyslexic strengths. Could you help me by sharing what you think I am good at? As I feel like years of criticism mean I only think about my dyslexic challenges'.

3. Start outside of work

If you're struggling to pinpoint your dyslexic strengths, start in your personal life, where there's often more space for them to shine.

For many dyslexics, anything to do with school or work carries a weight of challenge and expectation, meaning strengths feel invalidated or unappreciated. That can make it hard to see your strengths clearly, especially when they don't fit the 'norms' of what you 'should' be able to do.

Instead, start by speaking to your friends and family. What do they notice about you? What do you naturally gravitate towards in your free time? These insights can start to help you identify your strengths, which you can then bring into other areas of your life.

> ### Real-world story
>
> I worked with a woman who was an accountant. She struggled with the detailed aspects of the role and had faced repeated difficulties in her job – including being let go. This had really crushed her confidence, to the extent that she kept saying, 'I don't think I have dyslexic strengths.'
>
> To explore this, we tried looking at her personal life and seeing what areas she felt she excelled at. She told me she spoke four languages! She learned them by seeing the patterns and making connections and found it easy to pick up smatterings of other languages.
>
> Learning a language is usually considered a dyslexic challenge but by approaching it through her strengths, she was able to learn easily and found it enjoyable.

4. 'I thought everyone thought like that'

One of the most important parts of discovering your dyslexic strengths is realising that your thinking is unique. Often the problem that plagues people is thinking those around you have the same insights and ideas. I think this is often rooted in the idea that something impressive and valuable should be 'hard' to achieve and our unique approach and thoughts comes so naturally that they can't possibly be dyslexic strengths. Instead they must be how others see the world. This goes back to my point of high-value and low-value tasks, trying to recategorise what is hard and easy from what society has decided.

I often know someone has truly embraced their dyslexic strengths when they say, 'I thought everyone thought like this.'

Here are a few common examples of people not realising their dyslexic strengths and assuming everyone thinks like them:

- A new idea pops into your head and you think, *Someone must have thought of that*, so you stay quiet.
- You realise something won't work but you think, *They must know something I don't*, so you say nothing – and your prediction comes true or, even worse, someone says the same thing you'd thought of six months earlier.
- You see a new approach but stay quiet because there 'must be a reason' it's done the current way – even though it seems completely illogical to you.

So an important part of recognising your dyslexic strengths is realising that those ideas are unique and valuable. The second you start to think, *Oh, people don't think like that*, you're on your way to success. You'll begin to value your insights and be able to reduce the frustration and exhaustion that come from only focusing on the challenges.

How companies can support dyslexic strengths

One of the biggest challenges dyslexic professionals face is being appreciated and valued for our strengths. Too often, people are promoted based on their ability to do their current job, not on their potential to succeed in the next one. For dyslexics, this can mean being judged on tasks that foreground their challenges rather than their strengths.

Instead, the promotion process needs to allow people to showcase the value they could bring to the next role – such as strategic thinking – rather than focusing on skills that may be considered dyslexic challenges.

1. Allow people to showcase their strengths

Last year, I worked with a client who came to me with one simple goal: to get promoted. His difficulty was that he was struggling with some of the day-to-day tasks associated with his current role, which was making people doubt his capabilities.

Our coaching focused on helping him build a case that discounted the areas he was struggling with and showcased his strengths. Here's how we achieved this and an example of how other workplaces can do the same:

Be clear on the requirements of the role and focus on them

First, we got a list of the required skills for the next role. Then, instead of focusing on the challenges in the current role, we looked for ways to demonstrate those required skills – either within his current responsibilities or through new projects.

His current role involved managing 20 partners. This demanded high levels of organisation and attention to detail – skills with which he struggled and that had previously been flagged as needing work. The cognitive load of dealing with these challenges made him feel like he was pushing his brain up a hill every day. However, they were also skills that wouldn't be required to such an extent in the future role.

Our approach was to map the organisational skills needed for the future role against the skills he had: project management experience and the ability to deliver concepts on time and on budget. This shift in approach allowed him to showcase his skills and build a role around what came naturally.

Allow people to showcase their skills beyond their role

What made this process easier was that the company allowed his role to develop outside the core responsibilities. He took on strategic projects that better suited his strengths – and achieved a long list of huge wins that had material benefit for the entire team.

These types of tasks would usually not be worked on by someone more junior in the team, but because he knew his strengths, he worked hard to foreground them and demonstrate what was possible and how his career should be built.

2. Take ideas from different team members

Often, I think that people feel that managing dyslexia successfully within an organisation requires wholescale change. This isn't usually the case, though some specific areas might require an overhaul. Sometimes, it's as simple and easy as senior members of the team being open and approachable to new ideas.

I hear time and again from dyslexic professionals who hold back their ideas and value because they're worried about how they'll be received by senior management. Creating a culture where ideas are welcomed, regardless of role or communication style, can unlock enormous value.

3. Bear with the challenges

Dyslexic strengths offer huge advantages and opportunity – but they also come with real challenges that can require support.

One concept I always return to is this: dyslexic individuals are worth 'bearing with'. When we're not spending all our time focusing on and stressing about our challenges, we have more time and capacity to focus on our strengths – and the results speak for themselves.

For example:

- Your colleague is reminded about a client dinner the day before, knowing sometimes they forget or write things down wrong. They show up and help them chew through a problem by offering a fresh perspective. Their strengths of perceptiveness and their ability to understand a problem are worth bearing with, and far outweigh the minor support required to help them turn up on time.

- Your colleague's emails have occasional spelling mistakes, but their closing rate is phenomenal. You can either spend time asking them to double-check every email or shift their client approach to phone calls, where their persuasive skills shine. They are worth bearing with because their strengths of connecting with and persuading people are far more valuable then their ability to write error-free emails.

15
Seeing the big picture

> **Chapter summary**
>
> **Why this chapter is important**
>
> The dyslexic strength of big-picture thinking informs many of the other strengths that come so naturally us. When you understand what big-picture thinking truly means, it becomes much easier to unlock those other strengths.
>
> **What you will learn**
>
> - What big-picture thinking is and why it's the root of many dyslexic strengths.
> - How other dyslexic strengths link to big-picture thinking.
> - How understanding big-picture thinking will help you dial up your dyslexic strengths.

Many dyslexic strengths – and the way we talk about them – are quite ethereal or difficult to pin down. That is why in this section I am going to go into detail to help you feel really clear on each dyslexic strength, so you can fully understand each one's value and how it may show up for you.

What it is: Big-picture thinking is the ability to easily see the overview or full picture of how multiple concepts interconnect. It's like having a wider field of vision – dyslexic people naturally think about and look at more elements.

How to picture it: Imagine sitting on a plane and looking down at the world. You see all the fields, cars and people moving around at once. You're not down in the field working on one specific area but looking down from the sky seeing all the fields and how the water systems and road networks interconnect across large areas.

My term: I like to call this 'strategic thinking'. It's similar to 'big-picture thinking' but it's easier to understand and, importantly, it resonates more clearly with employers and has a much stronger perceived value.

Real-life examples of big-picture thinking

There isn't a single 'right' job for dyslexic thinkers – but in any role, this strength adds value.

Big-picture thinking in different careers and situations

The following are just a few brief examples of what big-picture thinking supports and allows in a range of different careers and scenarios:

- **Nursing** – spotting consistent problems on a ward and identifying policy changes that improve efficiency or recovery rates.
- **Teaching** – explaining the same concept in different ways to different children, thanks to having a good overview of the topic and flexible thinking.
- **Marketing** – having the overview of the market, which means it's easier to see market trends and come up with new ways to implement these with individual clients.
- **Consulting** – translating ideas across different clients or sectors and adapting concepts to suit different industries.

- **Office work** – identifying inefficiencies in systems and finding better methods that will save time and might lead to company-wide improvements.
- **Personal life** – many dyslexic individuals are known for giving insightful advice. This strength unlocked the door for me to understand and value my own dyslexic strengths, which is why I often tell my clients to start here, too.

How to explain big-picture thinking to others

Because terms like 'dyslexic strengths' and 'big-picture thinking' can seem vague, and may be confusing or awkward to explain, it's often easier to describe the *results* rather than the skills themselves. Instead of trying to explain skills, just highlight what you find easy and what it has achieved.

What to say to your boss

- 'I find it easy to spot potential gaps or problems in new projects because I like to understand how things work before moving forwards.'
- 'I enjoy identifying trends and thinking about solutions or new offers that might be beneficial. In the past this has led to big financial gains for my team.'
- 'I often draw insights from other industries or experiences, as I naturally spot similarities.'
- 'It's important to me to really understand a topic well, as it makes me feel clear on how to bring value to a task or what the best next step is.'
- 'In the past, I've become the go-to person to ask where to look for things or what we did previously, because I enjoy understanding the process and how things fit together.'
- 'People often say I'm good at seeing the truth of the situation – I cut through the fluff and get to the root of an issue.'

What to say to your friends, family or partner

- 'I really enjoy discussing perspectives or reasonings behind things – going to that deeper level of understanding helps me feel more confident.'
- 'If you explain to me why you want to do something or why you acted in that way, I find it easier to understand and process it.'
- 'I love understanding a problem from all angles and discussing ideas.'

How to build up the big picture

One of the realities of managing dyslexia is that when we don't have the big picture we are not able to access effective thinking and can feel confused or unsure about what to do next. But more importantly, it will feel like you're unable to access your dyslexic strengths. Whenever clients tell me they don't think they have this strength or feel like they are struggling to access that strength, my first question is: 'Do you have a full grasp of the big picture?'

This is why learning how to build up your big picture is important. This was also discussed in chapter 12, but here are a few more examples:

Strategies for individuals

1. Brain dump

This technique is essential for all dyslexic people. We need to get all the interconnections and thoughts that feel relevant out of our heads. Even if the links feel faint and don't fully connect yet, getting everything down first allows patterns and themes to build. A brain dump also helps you identify gaps and fully understand a problem. This is why mind-mapping (*see* p. 189) is such a powerful tool for dyslexics.

2. Create an overview

Our brains crave simplicity. Creating a clear overview allows you to connect all the individual details more easily. Starting with an overview is always helpful but if that isn't possible, begin with a simple explanation and then build up from there. This scaffolding helps reduce overwhelm and supports clarity.

3. Get more information

Dyslexic people are told repeatedly that we struggle with learning new topics – so it can be easy to think we need *less* information to process. But often, context and understanding the *why* behind a problem are essential for building up the big picture. Here are some questions I recommend asking:

- 'What was the reason behind that decision?'
- 'Is there any background that might be useful to understand?'
- 'Can you explain this with an example?'

4. Ensure you have a degree of autonomy

In my experience, dyslexic people who succeed have an element of autonomy in their role. Fixed structures and approaches don't always work well for us, especially when our instinct is to understand the process or improve the system.

When we are allowed to start from the beginning, learn everything and then build the project ourselves, at our own pace, we enjoy the challenge. We build up the big picture and then create the plan.

But if you're handed a process without explanation or context, it may not connect. If you can create autonomy in your role – even in small ways – you might find the big picture comes more naturally.

Examples of how to use big-picture thinking

Big-picture thinking isn't just a strength – a lot of the time it can be the way we think through tasks to make them easier. When creating strategies with clients, I often help them figure out how they can get that overview or big picture first and then build their process around it. This allows them to work *with* their brain, making tasks feel more manageable and intuitive.

Here are two examples of how my clients have done this:

Case study: primary school teacher

One of my clients is a primary school teacher who struggled with lesson planning and preparing all the topics across the 10 subjects covered. He constantly felt overwhelmed and could only focus on the immediate week's lessons, not the full term.

My first question was, 'How do you see the big picture of the task?' We quickly realised that he couldn't get 'up and out' of what was in front of him and see the bigger picture of the entire term.

So, we broke each subject down and assigned topics to specific weeks. This created a clear visual overview so he could see what needed to be done and when. This big picture helped him plan proactively rather than reactively and reduced his sense of overwhelm.

Visual overview example:

Week	Learning objective	Lessons that week
Week 1	Fractions	3
Week 2	Fractions	2
Week 3	Percentages	4
Week 4	Percentages	3

> **Case study: lawyer**
>
> Another client is a solicitor who constantly needs to quickly get up to speed with new cases. She was finding the process of digesting the information difficult and connecting all the details impossible in the time periods expected.
>
> We realised that instead of trying to learn everything at once, she needed to focus on getting the big picture first and then the details.
>
> We created a simple document to help her build the overview and see everything in one place. It asked three questions:
>
> 1. What is the case about?
> 2. What legal concepts are relevant?
> 3. What further information is needed?
>
> Focusing on the big picture allowed her to process the cases efficiently and then build up the details afterwards, without missing key elements.

The strengths that link to big-picture thinking

As I mentioned above, big-picture thinking lies at the root of many valuable dyslexic strengths. Here's how they connect, and how to understand them better:

Pattern recognition

What it is: The ability to notice when something becomes a theme and being able to pull trends from that pattern.

How it links to big-picture thinking: Seeing the overview and the connections makes the pattern obvious.

What it isn't: Being a mathematical genius. Patterns aren't just about numbers.

Explain it in a fun way: Your friend tells you about the new man she is dating and you realise they are suspiciously similar to the last. You can say to your friend, 'That is your type because of XYZ.'

Important fact: Pattern recognition and idea generation often arrive together. This is a great example of how some things come easily for us. We don't just spot the pattern – we instantly see what to do with it.

Examples:
- Identifying trends and building new offers.
- Recognising issues based on previous patterns.
- Always knowing who the killer is on detective shows.
- Knowing when your friend is upset even when they say they are fine, because you've learned their patterns.

The flip side: We don't enjoy information in isolation – we need to build up the big picture.

How companies can harness it: Create environments where any idea can come from any level of the business. Those closest to a problem often spot the problems or patterns first.

Problem-solving

What it is: Being met with a problem or situation and instantly coming up with five solutions, then quickly evaluating them and deciding which ones will or won't work.

How it links to big-picture thinking: Seeing all the parts of a problem makes it easier to find a route forwards.

What it isn't: Not every idea is gold-plated – us dyslexics haven't yet figured out how to achieve world peace.

Explain it in a fun way: You can think on your feet with daily challenges because you can see all the options. For example, I often forget important items when going on holiday or to festivals, but I can always think of a creative solution to get me out of this problem (including once forgetting my ticket to a gig!).

Important fact: It's not just the number of ideas but the ease with which they come to you.

Example: When you realise you forgot something important as you are walking to a festival, and then you have five different ideas about what to do.

The flip side: A lot of dyslexic people struggle with overwhelm – we see so many options and ways forward that choosing a path can feel difficult.

How companies can harness it: Allow time to break down problems and build an overview – making solutions easier to find.

Being an ideas person

What it is: Being able to have a conversation and come up with suggestions or options on how to move a concept forwards.

How it links to big-picture thinking: Our big-picture thinking means we are able to connect concepts together that others can't, allowing ideas from other industries or situations to be utilised.

What it isn't: Needing to have an idea or thought in *every* situation – you don't always have the understanding of a topic or the big picture to create the connections!

Explain it in a fun way: Isaac Newton is thought to have been dyslexic and I always feel like my ideas come to me like that apple dropping on his head – they just fall out of nowhere and it all clicks.

Example: People come to you to discuss problems or issues because they know you're likely to have a perspective or idea that could help them.

The flip side: It can make staying consistent on your own projects or work difficult, as there's always a new idea to distract you.

How companies can harness it: Use stories or examples to bring a situation to life and create better opportunities for ideas to flow.

Having a bullshit laser

What it is: Seeing through how someone explains something to determine the truth of the situation or what is likely to actually happen.

What it isn't: Having a fresh perspective or deeper thought in every situation – sometimes there's nothing to uncover.

Explain it in a fun way: Your friend tells you about a situation and how exciting it is but you see through it and realise it won't end well.

Examples:
- Spotting when people are being fake.
- Seeing through corporate fluff.

The flip side: When we don't understand a situation fully this fluff can distract us from the reality of what is being discussed and make processing harder.

How companies can harness it: Encourage clarity and transparency – dyslexic thinkers do best when they can cut through noise and see what matters.

Simplifying

What it is: Dyslexic people struggle with large amounts of information and like to get to the root of an issue, which means we can be great at boiling down a topic.

How it links to big-picture thinking: Seeing what is important and what isn't, so we can explain the overview of a topic well.

What it isn't: Learning something and straight away being able to explain it simply; you need to really know a topic to do this.

Explain it in a fun way: When you are listening to someone else explain a topic you know well and feel confused about why they've made it unnecessarily complex – you come in and explain it much more simply.

Examples:
- Being the go-to person for providing explanations.
- Building trust with people because they like your summaries.
- Constantly cutting slides, as simplicity matters.

The flip side: Too much information can overwhelm you, as you crave simplicity.

How companies can harness it: Letting people build up the big picture, so they feel confident enough to create the simplicity in their head. It might mean a few extra questions, but it will save time in the long run.

Why the big picture sucks sometimes

Listen, no one said that dyslexic strengths can't be annoying sometimes. But understanding the limits of your strengths helps you see their value. When you understand that a strength can still exist even if it's attached to a challenge, this can actually help the strength become more visible. Here's the flip side of big-picture thinking:

1. **Asking questions can feel embarrassing**
   Sometimes meetings or situations don't allow for questions, or the person you are working with is busy – and taking up their time to ask questions feels awkward.

2. **Details matter to others**
   Our focus is always on the big picture, which makes seeing the details difficult. In certain situations or for some people, that's

a problem. It doesn't make you 'less than' in some way – it just means that in those situations you need more support.

It is often the case that people who are good with detail don't see the big picture easily, so they may struggle with exactly what you find easy.

3. **It can be frustrating**
   Struggling to understand something often stems from an overwhelming amount of detail and a lack of overview. Knowing this doesn't make the frustration any less real.

4. **What's obvious to us isn't obvious to everyone**
   Explaining unique ideas can be painful and intimidating – especially to people more senior than us or sceptical peers. This adds to the frustration in struggling to communicate a point that feels so obvious to us but nobody else seems to get.

How companies can support big-picture thinking

1. Provide space to think

Position whiteboards in desk areas, not just meeting rooms, to allow for thought dumping and visual mapping.

Breakout spaces or quiet zones help dyslexic (and many other!) employees step out of the noise to focus and access strategic thinking. Extra points if you are on hand to talk through an idea or thoughts to help gain clarity and create connections faster.

2. Ensure employees aren't overloaded

When someone is bogged down handling emails or checking a document, they can't access higher thinking. If you overload a dyslexic person, they won't be able to step 'up and out' of the mundane tasks to access this thinking more consistently.

3. Provide context

A lot of companies are not interested in explaining *why* something is the case – they just expect people to blindly follow instructions. But providing the background can be really beneficial, especially if that context can be explained with stories or examples.

4. Clarify the overview first

Chunk and define topics rather than just pelting information at employees. Give a roadmap before diving into the details – this clear scaffolding is imperative for processing.

5. Follow up after delivering verbal information

Working memory challenges mean verbal-only instructions can be hard to retain. A dyslexic person will likely be focusing on getting down the key points and understanding what is being said and might miss some details. Follow-up notes allow dyslexic thinkers to listen and engage fully to see the connections, then focus on the detail in the notes at their own pace afterwards.

16
Understanding dyslexic strengths beyond big-picture thinking

> **Chapter summary**
>
> **Why this chapter is important**
>
> Dyslexic strengths are often complicated – wrapped in abstract terms that don't always readily make a lot of sense. Simplifying them is essential to really understanding your value and knowing where to focus.
>
> **What you will learn**
>
> - How to think about dyslexic creativity and image-centric thinking if you aren't naturally creative.
> - How to think about dyslexic strengths beyond having good ideas.
> - What 3D thinking is and why we need to value it as a dyslexic strength.

Understanding dyslexic creativity

Dyslexia is often linked to creativity – maybe for you that means you enjoy or are good at art, music or graphic design. It could be that this really resonates with you and you find designing your house or cultivating a style really enjoyable.

But for many, dyslexic creativity doesn't come easily or show up in traditional ways. Feeling like you have many dyslexic challenges but don't have one of the classic dyslexic strengths can be frustrating.

Other people feel their brain was made for creative work yet find themselves boxed into corporate roles or a life that doesn't seem like it was built for them.

This section helps you see dyslexic creativity beyond the usual expectations – and recognise the value it could have in other areas of your life.

Having a vision of how something will look

Dyslexic people often focus on images or have a picture in their mind's eye of how something might go. This visual representation can help us be creative. Here are a few examples:

- Designing visually engaging presentations.
- Focusing on branding because you understand the power of imagery.
- Explaining concepts by drawing them out – making ideas more engaging for others.
- Coming up with innovative ways to arrange and decorate your house or organise your space – this is especially useful for planning birthday parties!
- Being inventive in the kitchen – instead of following a recipe, which you might struggle to read, you visualise what you want to achieve and find your own method.

Being creative at explaining

Dyslexic people are excellent communicators and build connections with people well. A big part of this is due to *narrative reasoning*. We explain through stories, analogies and images, which makes our communication style more engaging and hooks people's interest.

> ### Case study: CMO of a major company
>
> I had a CMO of a large global company come on my podcast who told me he starts every Monday team meeting with a photo representing his priority for the week. Instead of explaining what he is working on using words, he shows an image that captures the concept. He feels this idea motivates his team to get behind the issue and helps them understand his priorities better. At the very minimum, the technique makes his Monday meeting more engaging.

Examples of dyslexic creative strengths

Narrative reasoning

What it is: Explaining and thinking through stories, images or analogies. This method helps people stay engaged for longer, builds trust and is persuasive.

What it isn't: Always needing to tell a story. Maybe you connect it to a TV show, a piece of music or a metaphor. These connections demonstrate our creativity and unique thinking.

Explain it in a fun way: You're not the boring person in a meeting – you bring the story that makes people engage.

Important fact: Explain things in the way *you* see them, not how you think others want to receive the information. Your natural narrative style is your strength and makes it easier for you to explain your ideas.

Example: I used to work in tech sales, selling an application programming interface (API) to companies. A lot of the people I needed to speak to before I got to the tech teams didn't understand what an API was or why it would help them. Part of my job was to explain it to them. I'd share stories of real problems and paint the picture – only then did my sales ability kick in. My brain naturally told stories, and that's what worked.

The flip side: Our stories can feel long-winded or tangential – but they're how we process and connect ideas.

How companies can harness it: Encourage creativity in how information is presented and allow dyslexics to take on persuading roles. It's important to provide context so that dyslexic employees are able to create connections that allow their strengths to shine.

3D thinking

What it is: Strong spatial skills – seeing physical items or concepts from every angle and mapping spaces or systems in your head. This dyslexic strength often gets less attention that it deserves, even though it's very valuable.

What it isn't: Seeing things this way all the time. It's a strength, not a constant state.

Explain it in a fun way: Walking around a city and instinctively knowing which direction you need to go, or being able to map out a city in your head once you have walked around it.

Important fact: If you want to be able to see every angle in your head and move it around – as people can with 3D thinking – you need to have all the information processed and a full understanding. If you haven't built up that understanding, 3D thinking is unlikely to happen.

Examples:
- Tradespeople who are dyslexic often say they are able to visualise alternative layouts or solutions because they 'see' the whole space and can move around it mentally.
- Dyslexic engineers describe their mind as being like a computer model – they can rotate and manipulate concepts internally.

The flip side: Seeing the overview of everything to do with a project or physical concept can make it difficult to see the details.

How companies can harness it: Providing tools to allow dyslexic employees to utilise this way of thinking, such as making sure there are whiteboards or the right software is available.

17
Dyslexic strengths in real life

> **Chapter summary**
>
> **Why this chapter is important**
>
> For many of us, the struggle of managing dyslexia has had a significant impact on our lives, causing low confidence, embarrassing mistakes and a huge dyslexic tax. Coming to terms with that and starting to find the silver lining in the challenges is an important part of the journey that will rebuild confidence and help you stand tall.
>
> **What you will learn**
>
> - The value of the dyslexic experience.
> - How to feel that hard work is a strength.
> - How to see the resilience of dyslexic people.
> - How to see the strength of dyslexic emotional awareness.

What is the dyslexic life experience?

If you think dyslexic strengths are just hard work then you are underestimating the value dyslexia can bring. Feeling proud about the value your dyslexic experience has given you is important, too. That is what we will be exploring here.

We've talked extensively about how dyslexic strengths are linked to how the brain processes information but many of us know that these strengths also come from our experiences. From school to work, we've learned the value of hard work and that if you struggle the first time it doesn't mean it's over – you can try again.

With so many people globally thought to be dyslexic, experiences inevitably vary. I have worked with people across the world, from the UK and Europe, US, across South America and Australia, and although there are differences in culture, there are also many commonalities.

Realising you're not alone and are tied to a wider collective experience is hugely important for helping you process and heal. It's also encouraging to acknowledge there are so many people out there using their dyslexic strengths in productive ways. So, here are some of the most common themes:

1. Accepting failure just means we need to try again

Dyslexic people don't always understand things the first time – whether it's learning to read or trying to pick up a card game on holiday. Whatever it is, the first time we try something, we often don't get the results we want. This of course applies for almost everyone, but most dyslexic people experience it more frequently and to a more significant degree.

This means that we learn early on that even when things don't go well the first time, we can pick ourselves up, dust ourselves off and try again. This is not easy – it may still feel embarrassing and you might even have to take a break before you feel confident to do it – but because we see repeatedly that if we try again, things work out, we understand how valuable it can be to keep going at a problem.

2. Consistent negative feedback

Dyslexia isn't about being stupid – but you often *feel* that way. You might have often experienced struggle or felt confused, and then there's the dreaded red pen across your work. This makes you feel like nothing you do is ever good enough or that no matter how hard you try, you will always face criticism.

I know this is something I used to dread in the workplace, after years of constantly feeling like I never achieved my potential at school. Each time I had an annual review and someone started to highlight my problems I would gear myself up for the emotions I would feel from being told I 'needed to double-check my work more'. It wasn't just about one criticism, but years and years of feedback or edits to my work.

One stat really helped bring this to life for me: experts estimate that children with ADHD receive 20,000 more negative messages by the age of 10 than their peers. While dyslexia is a different form of neurodivergence, you can get a sense of the scale of criticism we face and how exhausting it can be.

Strengths from the dyslexic experience

Despite the challenges dyslexic people face, these experiences feed into three powerful strengths I see across all my clients:

1. We are hard-working

If you ask a dyslexic person what their strengths are, a lot of the time they will tell you how hard-working they are. It's something to be hugely proud of and is noticed by others around us.

When hard work is drilled into you from a young age, you know that you can work through tough situations and are ready to roll up your sleeves and get started. What I like to remind people is our 'normal' is often 120 per cent, and we don't always realise how much effort we are actually putting in because going above and beyond is our standard a lot of the time.

This trait is often found in people who have their own businesses, which requires determination, perseverance and grit. However, it is also something that has huge benefits in many areas of life. It's important to realise that being someone who is willing to put in extra effort or hard work is noteworthy and noticed. One of my clients is the head of HR for a major international company and she often reflects on how her hard work ethic – due to her dyslexia – is one of the traits that mean her colleagues support and connect with her; they respect her determination, resilience and hard work. As she said: 'people commit to the committed.'

Sometimes we don't even realise all the ways this hard work is appreciated – it may not be said directly to us, but it is likely being said *about* us when we're being recommended to others.

Real-world story

As I mentioned earlier, I've had my probation extended many times in my career. Each time, I went into hyperdrive – working later, going above and beyond to try to upskill in the areas mentioned as being cause for concern. I often also took courses outside of work to improve my challenges.

In most cases, it wasn't the improvements I made that would get me off my performance plan, it was the *effort* and *hard work* I had put into managing my challenges that people would remark on and commend.

2. We are determined and resilient

As discussed previously, resilience and brushing yourself off and trying again is a core dyslexic strength. This occurs in all areas of life and a common example that comes up a lot is learning to drive.

Many dyslexic people struggle to pass their test and have to retake it multiple times. But they keep trying over and over again and eventually succeed.

That resilience is also what pushes us further in our careers and lives and helps us cope with life's hard knocks. It keeps us moving forwards to get to the next level and prove our capabilities.

When you listen to stories shared by people who are successful and who are talking about their dyslexia, and how it helped them, it is often this area of life – their determination and resilience – that they credit as helping them achieve more than many thought was possible for them.

3. We are emotionally intelligent

Dyslexia means you've likely had a lot of experience of struggling or feeling inadequate. That stays with you and makes you more aware of others who feel the same, creating a deep connection that drives you to want to make change to ensure it doesn't happen again. This can show up as:

- Being kinder to the new person who joins and taking time to explain to them topics that felt confusing for you.
- Having empathy when someone makes a mistake and trying to help them rectify it.
- Not judging when somebody finds something difficult and taking the time to help build a process rather than shaming them.

> **Real-world story**
>
> I've heard hundreds of examples of dyslexic people deciding to redo their companies' onboarding programmes, because they have struggled or been confused by the way the information was presented and want to ensure the next person doesn't feel the same way. So much so that I recently found myself laughing a little unprofessionally when a client told me that they had redone their company new starter pack – they had no idea that it was the third time I had heard that sort of story that week.

Why value these strengths?

Our dyslexic experiences and the strengths they have brought are often the key that has unlocked much of our success. The values of hard work, determination and empathy have driven us from a young age and pushed us beyond what might otherwise have been possible. They are a core part of being dyslexic – and when valued, they can truly be harnessed.

It's important when it comes to understanding and appreciating your dyslexic strengths to realise that they are unique to you. Don't undervalue or minimise them. Thanks to our challenges and lack of confidence, it's all too easy to dismiss them and shrug them off. Instead, make sure you acknowledge and appreciate the comments and compliments you get rather than just believing that anything that goes well is just 'a fluke'.

The reason this matters is that the more we put attention and focus on our strengths, the more we are able to use them and call on them.

What are the limitations of these strengths?

For all that they are hugely beneficial, it's important to recognise where dyslexic strengths have limits. This is especially true for our determination and hard work. These traits can be a double-edged sword – hard work is what has propelled us forwards but it's also what can be our downfall, leading to cycles of boom and bust, or big burnouts.

This particularly applies when we're working on something challenging without any dyslexic strategies, pushing ahead without any support – when getting help or doing things differently could make the process easier.

This doesn't mean that our strengths of hard work and determination aren't incredibly valuable and worth appreciating. But like all tools, they need to be considered carefully – knowing when to deploy them and how to use your resources responsibly.

Something to bear in mind is that hard work is now only one tool in your toolkit that you will carry into the future – a future that hopefully will now seem more positive, manageable and exciting.

Final thoughts: dyslexia is a journey, not a destination

The goal of this book was to help adults with dyslexia realise that there is a path through – and that simple strategies can make managing dyslexia successfully feel possible, maybe even easy. My hope is that next time someone is struggling, they won't have to wade through advice meant for children but instead can develop confidence, have strategies and unlock strengths.

The truth of managing dyslexia is that it's often a journey, not a destination. I believe there is no such thing as 'overcoming' dyslexia – instead, it's about accepting being different, working *with* your brain rather than against it, and trying to build a life around what you *can* do, not what you find exhausting. Most importantly, I want you to feel capable to do whatever you want in life and that dyslexia will never again make you shrink.

Thank you so much for taking the time to read this book. The strategies and advice shared have been a huge journey for me personally as I was always my first client. My story started with being unable to write full sentences and now I am a published dyslexic author. I feel my whole life has changed in a way I never thought possible and I'm so excited for the journey you will now go on with your dyslexia, too.

Acknowledgements

To my amazing mum, who from the very beginning valued my education and was determined to help me achieve my potential. You never stopped believing in me and telling me how incredible my brain was.

Thank you for all the hours you spent arguing with teachers, doing extra work with me and checking through my writing for spelling errors. Most of all, thank you for pointing out how my dyslexia made me exceptional at every turn and for never backing down when I dismissed you.

It took me years to believe everything you said about me, but I am so glad you persisted because I finally see what you see. This book and all of my work with Dyslexia in Adults is a testament to your commitment to me and my brain.

You believed in me when I didn't and you showed me I could when I thought I couldn't.

References

Introduction

'Dyslexia is a form of neurodivergence that affects an estimated one in 10 people': https://www.bdadyslexia.org.uk/dyslexia

Chapter 2, Dyslexic traits

'The 11 executive functions': https://dyslexiaida.org/executive-function-strategies-the-building-blocks-for-reading-to-learn/

'Approximately 25–40 per cent of individuals with dyslexia also meet diagnostic criteria for ADHD': Banfi, C., Landerl, K. and Moll, K. 'Cognitive Profiles and Co-occurrence of Dyslexia and Dyscalculia'. In: Skeide MA, ed. *The Cambridge Handbook of Dyslexia and Dyscalculia*. Cambridge Handbooks in Psychology. Cambridge University Press; 2022:65-82

'Around 40–50 per cent of children diagnosed with dyslexia show signs of dyscalculia': Ibid.

'30–50 per cent of people with dyslexia also experience motor coordination difficulties consistent with dyspraxia': Hollomotz, A., Priestley, M. and Andre, D., 'The lived experience of disabled people in the UK: a review of evidence', 17 July 2025. Available at: https://www.gov.uk/government/publications/the-lived-experience-of-disabled-people-in-the-uk-a-review-of-evidence/the-lived-experience-of-disabled-people-in-the-uk-a-review-of-evidence

Chapter 4, How to grow in confidence

'Under the Equality Act 2010': https://www.gov.uk/guidance/equality-act-2010-guidance

Chapter 6, How to get the most out of the strategies

'a habit takes around 60 repetitions to feel natural': https://pmc.ncbi.nlm.nih.gov/articles/PMC11641623/

Chapter 8, Tiredness

'...dyslexic people typically show reduced activity in the left hemisphere of the brain, which handles language and reading': Vain, Claire, 'Dyslexia Demystified: Understanding the Neurological Basis', May 2025. Available at: https://cpdonline.co.uk/knowledge-base/mental-health/dyslexia-demystified-understanding-neurological-basis/

'People with ADHD may have different circadian rhythms and work better later in the day': https://www.frontiersin.org/journals/psychiatry/articles/10.3389/fpsyt.2025.1697900/full

Chapter 9, Working memory

'Everyone (not just neurodiverse people) has a limited working memory capacity': Made by Dyslexia via, https://www.youtube.com/watch?v=KFdvzzkr6Vo

Chapter 17, Dyslexic strengths in real life

'...experts estimate that children with ADHD receive 20,000 more negative messages by the age of 10 than their peers': https://www.additudemag.com/children-with-adhd-avoid-failure-punishment/

For more information about Dyslexia in Adults, please scan the QR code.